Progress in Inflammation Research

Series Editor

Prof. Dr. Michael J. Parnham
PLIVA
Research Institute
Prilaz baruna Filipovica 25
10000 Zagreb
Croatia

(Already published titles see last page.)

Disease-modifying Therapy in Vasculitides

Cees G. M. Kallenberg
Jan W. Cohen Tervaert

Editors

Birkhäuser Verlag
Basel · Boston · Berlin

Editors

Cees G. M. Kallenberg
Department of Clinical Immunology
University Hospital Groningen
P.O. Box 30.001
9700 RB Groningen
The Netherlands

Jan W. Cohen Tervaert
Department of Clinical and Experimental Immunology
University Hospital Maastricht
P.O. Box 5800
6202 AZ Maastricht
The Netherlands

A CIP catalogue record for this book is available from the Library of Congress, Washington D.C., USA

Deutsche Bibliothek Cataloging-in-Publication Data
Disease modifying therapy in vasculitides / Cees G. M. Kallenberg ; Jan W. Cohen Tervaert,
ed.. - Basel ; Boston ; Berlin : Birkhäuser, 2001
    (Progress in inflammation research)
    ISBN 3-7643-6147-6

ISBN 3-7643-6147-6 Birkhäuser Verlag, Basel – Boston – Berlin

© 2001 Birkhäuser Verlag, P.O. Box 133, CH-4010 Basel, Switzerland
Member of the BertelsmannSpringer Publishing Group
Printed on acid-free paper produced from chlorine-free pulp. TCF ∞
Cover design: Markus Etterich, Basel
Cover illustration: Necrotizing crescentic glomerulonephritis as shown histologically (upper part) being one of the most important manifestations of small-vessel vasculitis associated with anti-neutrophil cytoplasmic antibodies (lower part). With friendly permission of C.G.M. Kallenberg.
Printed in Germany
ISBN 3-7643-6147-6

9 8 7 6 5 4 3 2 1   www.birkhauser.ch

Contents

List of contributors

Paul A. Bacon, Department of Rheumatology, Division of Immunity and Infection, University of Birmingham, Edgbaston, Birmingham, England, B15 2TT; e-mail: p.a.bacon@bham.ac.uk

Rainer Birck, Medizinische Klinik, Nephrologie/Endokrinologie, Universitäts- klinikum Mannheim, Theodor-Kutzer-Ufer 1–3, 68167 Mannheim, Germany

Maarten M. Boomsma, Department of Internal Medicine, Division of Clinical Immunology, University Hospital Groningen, 9713 GZ, Groningen, The Nether- lands; e-mail: M.M.Boomsma@INT.AZG.NL

David M Carruthers, Department of Rheumatology, City Hospital NHS Trust, Dud- ley Road, Birmingham B18 7QH, UK; e-mail: david.carruthers@cityhospbham.wmids.nhs.uk

Jan W. Cohen Tervaert, Department of Clinical Immunology, University Hospital Maastricht, P.O. Box 5800, 6202 AZ Maastricht, The Netherlands; e-mail: jw.cohentervaert@immuno.unimaas.nl

Loïc Guillevin, Department of Internal Medicine, Université Paris-Nord, Hôpital Avicenne, Assistance Publique – Hôpitaux de Paris, 125, rue de Stalingrad, 93009 Bobigny cedex, France; e-mail: loic.guillevin@avc.ap-hop-paris.fr

Ernst C. Hagen, Eemland Ziekenhuis, Locatie "Lichtenberg", Dept. of Internal Medicine, Utrechtsweg 160, 3818 ES Amersfoort, The Netherlands

Gary S. Hoffman, Department of Rheumatic and Immunologic Diseases, The Cleve- land Clinic Foundation / A50, 9500 Euclid Avenue, Cleveland, Ohio, 44195, USA

David Jayne, Department of Renal Medicine, Addenbrooke's Hospital, Cambridge CB1 2SP, UK; e-mail: dj106@cam.ac.uk

Cees G.M. Kallenberg, Department of Clinical Immunology, University Hospital Groningen, P.O. Box 30.001, 9700 RB Groningen, The Netherlands; e-mail: c.g.m.kallenberg@int.azg.nl

Carol A. Langford, National Institutes of Health, Building 10, Room 11B-13, Bethesda, MD, 20892, USA

Wilhelm H. Schmitt, Fifth Department of Medicine, University Hospital Mannheim, University of Heidelberg, Theodor Kutzer Ufer 1–3, 68167 Mannheim, Germany; e-mail: whschmit@rumms.uni-mannheim.de

Coen. A. Stegeman, Department of Internal Medicine, Division of Nephrology, University Hospital Groningen, Hanzeplein 1, 9713 GZ Groningen, The Netherlands; e-mail: C.A.Stegeman@int.azg.nl

John H. Stone, The Johns Hopkins Vasculitis Center, 1830 E. Monument Street, Suite 7500, Baltimore, Maryland 21205, USA; e-mail: jstone@welch.jhu.edu

Fokko J. van der Woude, Fifth Department of Medicine, University Hospital Mannheim, University of Heidelberg, Theodor Kutzer Ufer 1–3, 68167 Mannheim, Germany; e-mail: woude@rumms.uni-mannheim.de

Preface

During the last two decades the detection of anti-neutrophil cytoplasmic autoantibodies (ANCA) in the idiopathic small vessel vasculitides has renewed interest in the vasculitides in general. New concepts on classification, diagnosis and pathophysiology of this group of serious diseases have been presented. This has also stimulated clinical research on the treatment of the vasculitides.

In the 1970s, the introduction of cyclophosphamide, given in addition to corticosteroids, greatly improved prognosis of the necrotizing vasculitides. It became clear, however, that this regimen, in the long term, has limitations due to severe side-effects associated with its use. In recent years, gained insights into the pathogenesis of the vasculitides as well as the availability of new and more specific immunomodulatory drugs have opened new ways for treatment.

In this volume current standard treatment of the vasculitides, with recent adaptations, as well as new and more specific interventions are presented by authors who are in the forefront of vasculitis research. The work presents up-to-date information on treatment of vasculitides for the practical clinician, as well as considerations for future therapy.

We are indebted to all the contributing authors. Their expert knowledge and experience in the field of vasculitis guarantees thoughtful and innovative approaches to the present and future treatment of vasculitis. We are also grateful for the excellent secretarial assistance of Mrs. Kiki Bugter.

We hope that this book may be useful to all those who are treating systemic vasculitis for the benefit of patients suffering from these serious diseases.

Cees G. M. Kallenberg
Jan W. Cohen Tervaert

Systemic vasculitides, an introduction

Cees G.M. Kallenberg[1] and Jan W. Cohen Tervaert[2]

[1]Department of Clinical Immunology, University Hospital Groningen, P.O. Box 30.001, 9700
RB Groningen, The Netherlands; [2]Department of Clinical and Experimental Immunology,
University Hospital Maastricht, P.O. Box 5800, 6202 AZ Maastricht, The Netherlands

Introduction

Vasculitis is a condition characterized by inflammation of blood vessels. Its clinical
manifestations are dependent on the localization and size of the involved vessels as
well as on the nature of the inflammatory process. Vasculitis can be secondary to
other conditions or constitute a primary, in most cases, idiopathic disorder. Underlying conditions in the secondary vasculitides are infectious diseases, connective tissue diseases, and hypersensitivity disorders. Immune complexes, either deposited
from the circulation or formed *in situ*, are involved, in many cases, in the pathophysiology of the secondary vasculitides. Those complexes are supposedly com-
posed of microbial antigens in case of underlying infectious diseases, autoantigens
in the connective tissue diseases, and non-microbial exogenous antigens in the
hypersensitivity disorders (Tab. 1). Although immune deposits can be demonstrated
in the involved vessel wall by direct immunofluorescence of biopsy material, the
specificities of the antigens and their corresponding antibodies have not been
demonstrated in most of the cases.

The primary vasculitides (Tab. 2) are idiopathic systemic diseases with a variable
clinical expression [1]. Histopathologically, fibrinoid necrosis of the vessel wall is
apparent [2]. With the exception of Henoch Schönlein purpura and cryoglobulinemia associated vasculitis, the lesions are characterized by paucity of immune
deposits, and the pathophysiology of vessel wall inflammation in those pauci-
immune conditions is far from clarified. In the 1980s, however, autoantibodies to
cytoplasmic constituents of myeloid cells were detected in patients with idiopathic
necrotizing small-vessel vasculitis [3] (Tab. 2). Those anti-neutrophil cytoplasmic
autoantibodies (ANCA), particularly those reacting with proteinase 3 and myeloperoxidase, were shown to be sensitive and specific for the aforementioned conditions [4]. This suggests that the autoantibodies are involved in the pathogenesis of
the associated diseases and positions those diseases within the spectrum of autoimmune disorders.

Disease-modifying Therapy in Vasculitides, edited by Cees G. M. Kallenberg and
Jan W. Cohen Tervaert
© 2001 Birkhäuser Verlag Basel/Switzerland

Table 1 - Secondary vasculitides: antigens presumably involved

Exogenous antigens		
microbial antigens	bacterial	streptococci
		staphylococci
		mycobacterium leprae
		treponema pallidum
		others
	viral	hepatitis B/C virus
		human immunodeficiency virus
		cytomegalovirus
		Epstein-Barr virus
		others
	protozoal	plasmodia
non-microbial antigens	heterologous proteins	
	allergens	
	drugs	
	tumor antigens (?)	
Autologous antigens	nuclear antigens (antinuclear antibodies)	
	immunoglobulin G (rheumatoid factor, cryoglobulins)	
	others	

Primary systemic vasculitis – classification and clinical presentation

As stated before, a diagnosis of vasculitis is based on the presence of inflammation of the vessel wall. When other underlying conditions (Tab. 1) or direct infection of the vessel wall, either contiguous or *via* the blood stream, have been excluded [5], the vasculitis is idiopathic or primary. The primary vasculitides are classified based on the size of the vessels involved, the histopathology of the lesions, and the presence of characteristic clinical symptoms. A classification scheme as well as definitions for the various vasculitic syndromes have been proposed by an International Consensus Group in 1993 [1] (Tab. 2). Those definitions were not intended to be used as diagnostic criteria although many practitioners today base their diagnosis on the so-called Chapel Hill Consensus Conference definitions. In clinical practice, however, many patients with histologically confirmed vasculitis do not fulfill those Chapel Hill definitions either because they present with incomplete or overlapping clinical syndromes, or because biopsies fail to demonstrate the pathognomonic lesions as described in the definitions. In order to classify patients with histologically or angiographically proven vasculitis the American College of Rheumatology

Table 2 - Primary vasculitides [1]

Large vessel vasculitis	Giant cell (temporal) arteritis
	Takayasu's arteritis
Medium-sized vessel vasculitis	Polyarteritis nodosa
	Kawasaki disease
Small vessel vasculitis	Wegener's granulomatosis*
	Churg Strauss syndrome*
	Microscopic polyangiitis*
	Henoch-Schönlein purpura
	Essential cryoglobulinemic vasculitis
	Cutaneous leukocytoclastic angiitis

associated with anti-neutrophil cytoplasmic autoantibodies.

(ACR) has developed sets of criteria for the various vasculitides that are mostly based on clinical signs and symptoms [6]. Also those ACR-criteria have their limitations in terms of sensitivity and specificity.

Large vessel vasculitides

According to the Chapel Hill definitions [1] the vasculitic process in the large vessel vasculitides is confined to the aorta and its major branches.

The most common form, particularly in the white population, is *giant cell arteritis* [7]. Its name is derived from the presence of many Langhans' giant cells in the lesions. Histopathologically, invasion of the vessel wall with macrophages, and, to a lesser extent, lymphocytes and plasmacells is seen. Giant cells are clearly present and the internal elastic membrane is disrupted. At some areas calcification of the internal elastic membrane with focal accumulation of giant cells only has been observed [8], and it has been suggested that those foreign body giant cells are secondary to degeneration of the internal elastic membrane. Next, an autoimmune response would ensue as those giant cells present degenerated membrane structures to T lymphocytes (see later). Clinically, the disease frequently presents with headache, tenderness of the scalp, particularly of the temporal arteries (which has led to the synonymous designation of temporal arteritis), and claudication of the jaws. In addition, symptoms related to ischaemia of arteries in the upper part of the body may be present, such as loss of vision due to vasculitis of the retinal artery and neurological defects due to vasculitis of the internal carotid artery, the vertebrobasilar artery, and

3

intracerebral arteries. Other systems may be involved as well. In addition, the syndrome of polymyalgia rheumatica consisting of pain and stiffness of the proximal extremities is present in about 50% of patients. Systemic symptoms such as fatigue, malaise and fever with highly elevated ESR and anemia are almost invariably present. The disease generally occurs at older age, above 50 years, almost exclusively in whites, with an incidence of 17 per 100,000 persons above 50 years.

Takayasu arteritis is a second form of large vessel vasculitis [9, 10]. It affects the aorta and its brachiocephalic branches but may also affect the pulmonary arteries, other visceral arteries, and the arteries of the lower extremities. Histopathologically, various stages may be present. Active lesions are characterized by a granulomatous giant cell arteritis with a lymphoplasmacytic infiltrate with eosinophils, histiocytes and Langhans' cells. As a result of active inflammation segmental narrowing and dilatation with aneurysm formation may occur histopathologically characterized by fibrosis and focal destruction of the musculoelastic layers. At the time of active inflammation systemic symptoms are present accompanied by an increased acute phase response. Later occurring symptoms are related to the localization and the extent of obstruction of the involved vessels and may include claudication of upper and lower extremities (so-called "pulseless" disease), cerebral symptoms, ischemic bowel disease, renovascular hypertension, aortic insufficiency, etc. The disease occurs at a younger age than with giant cell arteritis, particularly in women between 15 and 45 years, is relatively rare with an incidence of 2–20 per million, and is more frequent in Orientals, Africans and Latin Americans.

Medium-sized vessel vasculitis

Classical *polyarteritis nodosa* (PAN), according to the Chapel Hill definitions [1], is a form of vasculitis confined to medium-sized arteries without involvement of smaller sized vessels [11]. Applying that definition, PAN is now a rare disease [12], and many cases formerly diagnosed as PAN are now classified as microscopic polyangiitis (see below). The disease is histopathologically characterized by fibrinoid necrosis of the vessel wall with, frequently, microaneurysm formation. Those microaneurysms can be visualized by visceral angiography and may be a clue to diagnosis.

Clinically, systemic symptoms including fever, fatigue, weight loss, arthralgia and myalgia are almost invariably present. Other symptoms are related to involvement of specific arteries such as renal insufficiency and malignant hypertension in case of renal vasculitis, ischemic bowel disease when the mesenteric arteries are involved, etc. The disease has been associated with Hepatitis B virus infection as well as with HIV-infection, albeit in a minority of the cases [13].

Another form of vasculitis of medium sized arteries is *Kawasaki syndrome*, also designated as mucocutaneous lymph node syndrome, a disease that particularly occurs in childhood [14]. The disease presents with fever, a polymorphous exanthema especially on the palms and soles, reddening of lips and oral cavity, bilateral conjunctival injection, and cervical lymphadenopathy. These symptoms suggest an infectious etiology but no specific microorganism has been identified. Analysis of the T-cell repertoire showed selective expansion of T cells expressing T-cell receptor variable regions Vβ2 and Vβ8 suggesting bacterial superantigen stimulation [15]. In some 35% of cases vasculitis of the coronary arteries occurs. The disease is most frequent in Japan where its incidence is 150 per 100,000 children under the age of five years.

Small vessel vasculitis

Within the spectrum of vasculitis, the idiopathic small vessel vasculitides, that is Wegener's granulomatosis, microscopic polyangiitis, and Churg Strauss syndrome, are strongly associated with the presence of anti-neutrophil cytoplasmic antibodies (ANCA) as will be discussed later on [4]. *Wegener's granulomatosis* (WG) is characterized by the triad of granulomatous inflammation of, particularly, the respiratory tract, systemic vasculitis, and necrotizing crescentic glomerulonephritis (Fig. 1) [16, 17]. Limited forms in which the kidney is not involved, may occur. The disease generally follows a biphasic course. Initially, inflammatory lesions of the upper respiratory tract occur, such as chronic sinusitis, rhinitis, and/or otitis, with ongoing destruction resulting, for example, in a saddle nose deformity. Systemic symptoms such as malaise, arthralgias and myalgias, are frequently present. Later on, systemic vasculitis with rapidly progressive glomerulonephritis develops in many patients. Other organs including the lungs (focal granulomatous vasculitic lesions that may cavitate), the eyes, the skin, and the peripheral nervous system are frequently involved as well. The disease occurs somewhat more frequently in white men, with an onset around the fifth decade, and has a higher incidence in northern countries. As in other vasculitides relapses frequently occur. Without treatment prognosis is poor with a mean survival of less than 6 months.

Microscopic polyangiitis (MPA) frequently presents as a renal-pulmonary syndrome with pulmonary capillaritis and necrotizing crescentic glomerulonephritis together with systemic symptoms such as fever, malaise, arthralgia and myalgia [11, 18]. In contrast to Wegener's granulomatosis granulomatous inflammation and/or destructive lesions of the upper respiratory tract are absent. Small vessel vasculitis is prominent whereas vasculitis in classical PAN is confined to medium sized arteries (see before). Besides lung- and kidney involvement, other organs such as eyes, skin and peripheral nervous system may be involved as well. A renal limited form has been described as idiopathic necrotizing crescentic glomerulonephritis. As in most of the idiopathic systemic vasculitides the lesions are characterized by absence or paucity of immune deposits. Age at onset and sex distribution are comparable to that in Wegener's Granulomatosis.

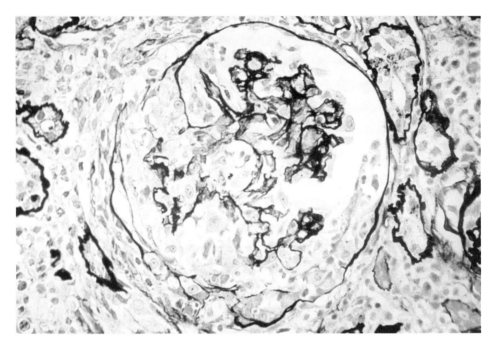

Figure 1
Lightmicroscopy of lesions found in a renal biopsy from a patient with Wegener's granulo-
matosis showing crescent formation, tuft necrosis, gaps in Bowman's capsule, and
periglomerular infiltration. Methamine-silver with aniline red counterstaining (original mag-
nification × 625).

Churg-Strauss syndrome (CSS) differs from WG and MPA by the presence of asthma and hypereosinophilia [13, 19]. Patients, generally, have a long history of asthma and hypereosinophilia (> 1500/mm^3) before they develop systemic vasculitis. Eosinophil-rich granulomatous inflammation occurs in the respiratory tract and clinically manifest as lung infiltrates and rhinitis with polyposis. Necrotizing vasculitis of small and medium-sized vessels with infiltration of eosinophils underlies the clinical manifestations of mononeuritis multiplex, ischemic bowel disease, and purpura or nodules of the skin. Renal involvement occurs less frequently than in WG and MPA. Cardiomyopathy, occurring in about 50% of the patients, is a major cause of mortality. The disease presents at the age of 35–40 years, equally in males and females.

Three other disease entities are included in the group of small vessel vasculitides according to the Chapel Hill classification. *Henoch-Schönlein purpura*, predominantly occurring in children, is clinically characterized by attacks of purpura, arthralgia/arthritis, and gastrointestinal symptoms [20, 21]. Glomerulonephritis occurs less frequently in children but is a frequent finding when Henoch-Schönlein purpura presents at older age. Skin and intestinal lesions are histopathologically characterized by leucocytoclastic vasculitis with IgA deposits in the vessel wall. Renal pathology varies from mesangial *via* focal-segmental to diffuse proliferative glomerulonephritis with sometimes also extracapillary proliferation. IgA deposits are primarily localized in the mesangium but may also be present in the capillary wall accompanied by C3 (but not C1q and C4) in most of the cases. Attacks frequently occur in association with (respiratory tract) infections but neither a causative agent nor a specific antigen have been identified. The disease, in most of the cases, is self limiting but proliferative glomerulonephritis may progress to end-stage renal failure.

Essential cryoglobulinemic vasculitis [13, 22, 23] is a form of immune complex mediated vasculitis. Circulating cryoglobulins consist of polyclonal IgG and monoclonal (type II) or polyclonal (type III) IgM with rheumatoid factor activity. IgG- and IgM deposits are detectable in the lesions. The disease is particularly associated with Hepatitis B- and C-virus infection. Clinically, purpura, arthralgia, and peripheral neuropathy are most prominent, whereas renal involvement is less common.

Cutaneous leukocytoclastic angiitis [24] in most cases is a form of secondary vasculitis. As discussed before immune deposits are present within the vessel wall. It may, however, occur as an idiopathic variety with paucity of immune deposits. As the therapeutic strategy for isolated cutaneous angiitis should be less aggressive than for the systemic vasculitides, cutaneous angiitis has been included in the Chapel Hill classification as a separate category [1].

Serological findings in the primary systemic vasculitides

As for the large vessel vasculitides, no disease-specific autoantibodies have been described until now. Also in medium-sized vessel vasculitis, specific autoantibodies are lacking. Anti-endothelial cell antibodies (AECA) have, however, been described in the primary vasculitides but also in secondary vasculitides, connective tissue diseases, and a variety of other (inflammatory) disorders [25]. AECA represent a heterogeneous group of antibodies and their target antigens are, generally, poorly characterized [25, 26]. AECA are generally detected by enzyme-linked immunosorbent assays (ELISA) using as a substrate cultured human umbilical vein endothelial cells (HUVEC) [25, 26]. AECA react with different endothelial antigens ranging in molecular weight from 25–200 kDa [25]. As stated, AECA frequently occur in the systemic vasculitides but are clinically of little value due to lack of disease specificity. Possibly, full characterization of the target antigens will improve their diagnostic significance. In this respect, AECA from a patient with Takayasu arteritis proved to react specifically with large vessel endothelial cells and activate those cells *in vitro* [27].

Anti neutrophil cytoplasmic antibodies (ANCA) were first described as sensitive and specific markers for active WG [3]. The autoantibodies in WG produce a characteristic cytoplasmic staining pattern (c-ANCA) by indirect immunofluorescence on ethanol-fixed neutrophils (Fig. 2). The target antigen of c-ANCA is proteinase 3, a third serine protease, besides elastase and cathepsin G, from azurophilic granules [28]. Shortly after the detection of c-ANCA in WG, it proved that many patients with related conditions, that is MPA, CSS, and idiopathic necrotizing crescentic glomerulonephritis (NCGN), had autoantibodies that produced a perinuclear staining pattern (p-ANCA) on ethanol-fixed neutrophils. The target antigen of p-ANCA in those conditions is myeloperoxidase (MPO) [4]. P-ANCA do, however, occur in many other conditions as well [4, 29]. The target antigens in those, generally inflammatory, conditions that differ from the idiopathic small vessel vasculitides, are very diverse and include lactoferrin, bactericidal permeability increasing protein, cathepsin G, and many other antigens, many of which are not yet characterized. It should be stated that only anti-PR3 and anti-MPO antibodies are currently of diagnostic significance in the primary vasculitides.

Three major studies on more than 200 patients have found a sensitivity of c-ANCA/anti-Pr3 of 90% for extended WG characterized by the triad of granulomatous inflammation of the respiratory tract, systemic vasculitis, and necrotizing crescentic glomerulonephritis [30–32]. The sensitivity of anti-Pr3 for limited WG, i.e. disease manifestations without obvious renal involvement, amounted to 75% [31]. Specificity of anti-Pr3 for WG or related small-vessel vasculitides was 98% when selected groups of patients with idiopathic inflammatory or infectious diseases were tested [30, 31]. The aforementioned studies were performed by groups highly experienced in ANCA-testing. The high sensitivity and specificity of cANCA for WG have, however, been questioned [33]. Rao et al. [34] did a meta-analysis on the role of cANCA testing in the diagnosis of WG. Summarizing current literature, they found a sensitivity of 66% and a specificity of 98% of c-ANCA for a diagnosis of WG. Sensitivity rose to 91% when patients with active disease only were considered. Anti-Pr3 also occurs in primary vasculitides other than WG: 25–40% of patients with MPA, 20–30% of patients with idiopathic necrotizing and crescentic glomerulonephritis (NCGN), and a minority of patients with CSS test positive for anti-Pr3 (reviewed in [4]). Anti-Pr3 has only very incidentally been reported in other disorders [4].

Figure 2

Staining of ethanol fixed neutrophils by indirect immunofluorescence by sera producing (A) a characteristic cytoplasmic staining pattern with accentuation of the fluorescence intensity in the area within the nuclear lobes (c-ANCA),
(B) a perinuclear staining pattern (p-ANCA).

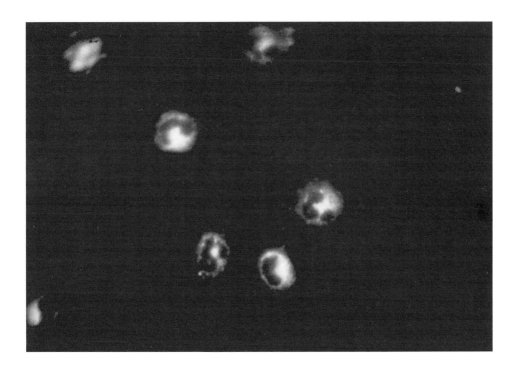

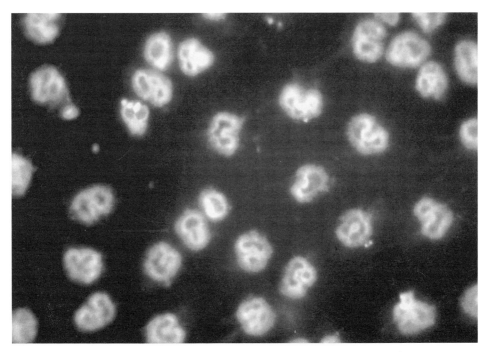

Whereas anti-Pr3 are primarily associated with WG, anti-MPO are found in primary vasculitis patients with a more diverse presentation [35, 36]. In WG, most of the patients who test negative for anti-Pr3, are positive for anti-MPO. Also, some 60% of patients with MPA, 65% of those with idiopathic NCGN, and 60% of those with CSS are positive for anti-MPO [34-36]. Anti-MPO have also been detected in 30–40% of patients with anti-GBM disease [37]. Furthermore, anti-MPO have been reported in connective tissue diseases such as SLE and in various drug-induced disease states such as hydralazine-induced glomerulonephritis, vasculitis-like syndromes associated with propylthiouracil, other antithyroid medications, minocycline and penicillamine (reviewed in [29]). In view of the poor specificity of pANCA as detected by IIF for the systemic vasculitides testing for ANCA in patients suspected of vasculitis should include tests for both anti-Pr3 and anti-MPO. A large-sized, prospective European collaborative study has, indeed, analyzed the sensitivity and specificity of anti-Pr3/anti-MPO for the idiopathic small vessel vasculitides [38]. This study found that the combination of cANCA by IIF and anti-Pr3 by ELISA or pANCA by IIF and anti-MPO by ELISA had a specificity of 98.4% in a group of 153 patients with either WG, MPA or idiopathic NCGN compared to 184 disease controls and 740 healthy subjects. In that multi-center study the sensitivity of cANCA + anti-Pr3 or pANCA + anti-MPO for WG, MPA or idiopathic NCGN was 73%, 67%, and 82%, respectively; these numbers are somewhat lower than in other studies, possibly since patients with minor disease activity were included as well.

In conclusion, anti-Pr3/anti-MPO, but not (p)ANCA alone, are highly specific and reasonably sensitive markers for the idiopathic necrotizing small vessel vasculitides.

Pathogenesis of the systemic vasculitides

Understanding the pathogenesis of the systemic vasculitides is important for the development of rational treatment modalities that specifically intervene with pathways in the etiopathogenesis of those diseases. Unfortunately, we know hardly anything of the etiology of the vasculitides and we are only in the beginning of the elucidation of their pathogenesis although particular pathophysiological pathways have been unraveled. As a result causal treatment is not yet possible and current treatment modalities are generally based on non-specific immunosuppression (see the chapter by Cohen Tervaert et al. in this volume). Nevertheless, advances have been made, recently, in the understanding of the pathophysiology of the ANCA-associated vasculitides as well as in giant cell arteritis.

What do we know about the pathophysiological role of ANCA in their associated conditions? As already discussed, ANCA directed to either MPO or PR3 are closely associated with pauci-immune necrotizing crescentic glomerulonephritis, either idiopathic or as part of WG, MPA and CSS [4]. Longitudinal observations point to a relationship between changes in level of the autoantibodies and changes in disease activity of the associated disorders. Rises in titres of ANCA appear to precede clinical disease activity [30] and treatment based on changes in ANCA titres resulted in the prevention of disease relapses [39]. These studies, generally based on small series of patients, used ANCA titration in the indirect immunofluorescence test for quantification, which, certainly, is not the most accurate way of quantitating levels of autoantibodies. Indeed, other authors could not confirm a strong correlation between rising titres and ensuing relapses [40]. Recently, Boomsma et al., in a 2-year prospective study, have analyzed this relationship in 85 patients with anti-PR3 associated glomerulonephritis/vasculitis using ELISA for quantification of the autoantibodies. They found that 27 out of the 33 relapses that occurred during the study period were preceded by a significant rise in PR3-ANCA levels, whereas 11 rises in PR3-ANCA occurred that were not followed by a relapse [41]. In addition to those data, it has been proven that patients with anti-PR3 associated disease have an eight-fold increased risk for development of a relapse once tests for ANCA are persistently or intermittently positive after induction of remission [42]. Taken together, all these *in vivo* data suggest that ANCA are involved in the pathophysiology of PR3-ANCA/MPO-ANCA associated pauci-immune glomerulonephritis. What other data are available to support a pathophysiological role for ANCA? *In vitro*, ANCA are able to activate neutrophils to the production of reactive oxygen species and the release of lytic enzymes such as elastase and PR3 [43]. In order to get activated by ANCA neutrophils must be in a state of pre-activation ("primed"). Priming occurs in the presence of low amounts of pro-inflammatory cytokines such as tumor necrosis factor-α (TNFα) or interleukin-1 (IL-1). During priming the target antigens of ANCA, that is PR3 and MPO, are expressed at the cell surface and, so, accessible for interaction with ANCA. This interaction followed by activation of neutrophils only occurs when neutrophils are adherent to a surface, a process in which β_2-integrins are involved [44]. *In vivo*, this process, thus, is assumed to occur at the endothelial surface. Indeed, activated neutrophils adherent to the endothelium are observed in renal biopsies from patients with ANCA-associated NCGN [45]. ANCA induced neutrophil activation involves not only binding of the antibodies *via* their $F(ab^1)_2$-fragments to surface expressed PR3 or MPO, but also interaction of their Fc-fragments with Fc-receptors on neutrophils, particularly with the Fcγ RIIa-receptor [46].

In vitro studies using endothelial monolayers also have shown that neutrophils, in the presence of ANCA are able to adhere to and lyse endothelial cells [47, 48]. Elegant studies by the group of Savage demonstrated that ANCA are able to induce stable adherence of rolling neutrophils to layers expressing adhesion molecules [49]. Whether endothelial cells themselves express ANCA-antigens such as PR3, has been a subject of controversy. Data from Mayet et al. suggest that endothelial cells express PR3, particularly when activated, and that, subsequently, ANCA can bind to surface expressed PR3 resulting in upregulation of adhesion molecules and further activation of those cells [50]. Others, however, have not been able to confirm PR3 expression by endothelial cells [51] but demonstrated that PR3 binds to endothelial cells *via* a specific receptor [52].

More definite evidence for a pathophysiological role of ANCA may come from animal models. Unfortunately, fully satisfactory models for ANCA-associated glomerulonephritis are not (yet) available. Passive transfer of ANCA in primates or inducing an autoimmune response to MPO in rats did not result in renal lesions [53]. When, however, the products of activated neutrophils, that is lytic enzymes, MPO, and its substrate H_2O_2, are perfused into the renal artery in rats immunized with MPO, severe pauci-immune NCGN develops [53]. The results of those studies suggest that, initially, cationic proteins, such as MPO and PR3, from activated neutrophils adhere to the glomerular capillary wall and are bound by their cognate antibodies. The *in situ* formed immune complexes activate the complement system resulting, amongst others, in attraction of neutrophils. Those neutrophils are subsequently activated by ANCA and degrade the immune complexes that were initially present. The potential of ANCA to augment *in vivo* an inflammatory reaction has been demonstrated by Heeringa et al. [54] in an animal model of anti-glomerular basement membrane (anti-GBM) disease. They injected a subclinical dose of heterologous anti-GBM antibodies in rats which resulted in deposition of immunoglobulins along the GBM but did not induce severe glomerulonephritis. In rats immunized with human MPO, which led to the development of anti-MPO antibodies cross-reacting with their own MPO, however, severe necrotizing and crescentic glomerulonephritis developed after injection of this subclinical dose of anti-GBM antibodies. These experiments most convincingly show the phlogistic potential of ANCA. Nevertheless, a fully satisfying animal model for ANCA-associated vasculitis/glomerulonephritis does not yet exist [55].

Taken together, there are strong indications that ANCA are involved in the pathophysiology of the associated glomerulonephritides but definite proof is lacking (Fig. 3).

Figure 3.

Schematic representation of the immune mechanisms supposedly involved in the pathophysiology of ANCA associated vasculitides.

(1) Cytokines released due to (local) infection cause upregulation of adhesion molecules on the endothelium and priming of neutrophils and/or monocytes. (2) Circulating primed neutrophils and/or monocytes express the ANCA antigens on the cell surface. (3) Adherence of primed neutrophils and/or monocytes to the endothelium, followed by activation of these cells by ANCA. Activated neutrophils and/or monocytes release reactive oxygen species (ROS) and lysosomal enzymes, which leads to endothelial cell injury and eventually to necrotizing inflammation. (4) Degranulation of proteinase 3 and myeloperoxidase by these ANCA activated neutrophils and/or monocytes results in endothelial cell activation, endo-

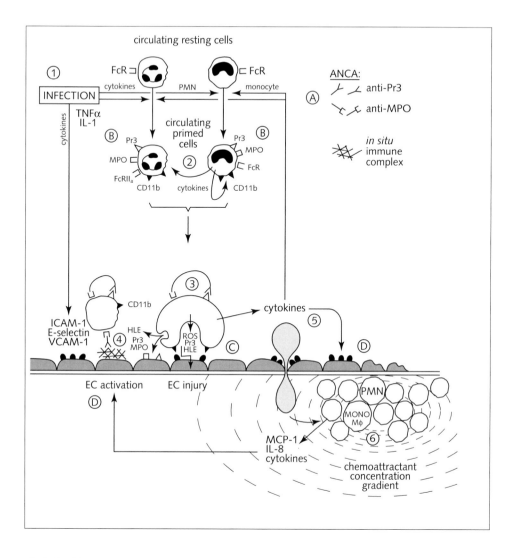

thelial cell injury or even endothelial cell apoptosis. Furthermore, bound Pr3 and MPO serve as planted antigens, resulting in in situ immune complexes, which in turn attract other neutrophils. (5) ANCA induced monocyte activation leads to production of monocyte chemoattractant protein-1 (MCP-1) and interleukin 8 (IL-8) production by these cells. The release of these chemoattractants by these cells amplifies monocyte and neutrophil recruitment possibly leading to granuloma formation (6). (A) to (D) represent the four prerequisites for endothelial cell damage by ANCA; (A) the presence of ANCA, (B) expression of the target antigens for ANCA on primed neutrophils and monocytes, (C) the necessity of an interaction between primed neutrophils and endothelium via β2-integrins, and finally, (D) activation of endothelial cells.

What do we know about the pathogenesis of giant cell arteritis, one of the most frequent systemic vasculitides? Giant cell arteritis (GCA), as discussed before, is a form of large vessel vasculitis generally occurring at older age. It is characterized by a granulomatous inflammatory reaction within the vessel wall with accumulation of T-cells, macrophages, and multinucleated giant cells. Its etiology is unknown but variations of incidence with grouping of cases in certain areas have suggested that environmental infections could play a role [56]. The predilection of the disease for white people from northern European countries and northern areas in the USA suggests that besides environmental also genetic factors are involved. HLA-typing has shown an association with HLA-DR4 and with HLA-DRB1 alleles, particularly with DRB*04 [57, 58] as in rheumatoid arthritis. This association was accompanied by corticosteroid resistance [58] suggesting a more severe variety of the disease which was, however, not confirmed in another study [57]. HLA associations may mechanistically be explained in different ways but point particularly to the involvement of antigen-specific T lymphocytes in the pathogenesis of the associated disorder. To further investigate the nature of the antigen-specific T-cell response in GCA, Martinez-Taboada et al. [59] analyzed the presence of clonally expanded T cells in biopsies from temporal arteries. By systematical screening of the T-cell receptor β chain repertoire from eight biopsies they found clonally expanded T cells in 30% of the βV-J combinations. Some of these clones were present at different sites in the biopsy but not in the peripheral blood. Sequencing showed a diversity of Vβ chain sequences. One of the T-cell clonotypes showed proliferation when incubated with monocytes pulsed with temporal artery extracts from patients but not with extracts from control temporal arteries. These data point to an (auto)antigen-specific T-cell response in which a modified antigen may be involved. In this respect actinically degenerated elastic tissue has been suggested as the relevant autoantigen [60] although characterization of the precise antigenic structures and their modification(s) has not been accomplished. Further proof for the role of T cells in the pathogenesis of GCA was obtained by implanting diseased temporal artery specimens from GCA patients into SCID mice in order to study the T-cell dependency of the lesions [61]. The inflammatory infiltrate persisted after implantation with expansion of certain T cells producing interleukin-2 (IL-2) and interferon γ (IFNγ) so inducing the production of IL-1β and IL-6 by monocytes/macrophages. The selective expansion of those T cells in the context of diseased arteries suggest a locally expressed antigen and an ensuing Th-1 type reaction.

Analysis of cytokine patterns in biopsies from patients with GCA also shows mRNA expression of IL-2 and IFNγ as well as IL-1β but not of IL-10 [62]. Interestingly, the presence of giant cells was associated with local synthesis of IFNγ. Thus, *in vivo* data from patient material also point to a Th-1 type of response in which macrophages are important effector cells. Those macrophages and multinucleated giant cells produce platelet-derived growth factor (PDGF) A and B [63] which might, at least in part, be responsible for intimal proliferation and luminal narrowing. Those activated macrophages also produce nitric oxide radicals and reactive oxygen species which, together, induce tissue damage by lipid peroxidation and peroxynitrite induced nitration of tyrosine residues on proteins [64].

In conclusion, T-cell based autoimmunity seems to underlie giant cell arteritis. Characterization of the relevant autoantigen(s) and epitopes, whether or not constitutive or modified proteins, is still a major challenge.

Conclusion

The primary systemic vasculitides constitute a group of clinically heterogeneous disorders characterized by idiopathic inflammation of the vessel wall. Classification, based on histopathological findings as well as clinical symptoms, is important in order to study clinical course, response to treatment, and outcome for the various disorders. Unfortunately, their etiopathogenesis has not been fully elucidated. Both exogenous, genetic, and, particularly, autoimmune factors seem to be involved in their pathogenesis. Autoimmune responses to myeloid lysosomal proteins, particularly proteinase 3 and myeloperoxidase, are involved in the pauci-immune small vessel vasculitides and a wealth of data now support their pathogenetic role. In large vessel vasculitides specific T-cell responses, possibly directed to modified vessel wall proteins, seem to underlie the disease process but, again, characterization of the target antigens is still lacking. Elucidation of the precise pathogenetic mechanisms will allow more specific treatment for this group of diseases which still have a high degree of morbidity and mortality.

References

1 Jennette JC, Falk RJ, Andrassy K, Bacon PA, Churg J, Gross WL, Hagen EC, Hoffman GS, Hunder GG, Kallenberg CG et al (1994) Nomenclature of systemic vasculitides. Proposal of an international consensus conference. *Arthritis Rheum* 37: 187–192

2 Lie JT (1989) Systemic and isolated vasculitis: a rational approach to classification and pathologic diagnosis. *Pathol Annu* 24: 25–114

3 Woude FJ van der, Rasmussen N, Lobatto S, Wiik A, Permin H, Es LA van, Giessen M van der, Hem GK van der, The TH (1985) Autoantibodies to neutrophils and monocytes: a new tool for diagnosis and a marker of disease activity in Wegener's granulomatosis. *Lancet* ii: 425–429

4 Kallenberg CGM, Brouwer E, Weening JJ, Cohen Tervaert JW (1994) Anti-neutrophil cytoplasmic antibodies: current diagnostic and pathophysiological potential. *Kidney Int* 46: 1–15

5 Somer T, Finegold SM (1995) Vasculitides associated with infections, immunization, and antimicrobial drugs. *Clin Infect Dis* 20: 101–136

6   Hunder GG, Arend WP, Bloch DA, Calabrese LH, Fauci AS, Fries JF, Leavitt RY, Lie JT, Lightfoot RW Jr, Masi AT et al (1990) The American College of Rheumatology 1990 criteria for the classification of vasculitis. Introduction. *Arthritis Rheum* 33: 1065–1067

7   Hunder GG (2000) Giant cell arteritis and polymyalgia rheumatica. *Clin Exp Rheumatol* 18 (4 Suppl 20): S1–S60

8   Nordberg E, Bengtsson BA, Nordberg C (1991) Temporal artery morphology and morphometry in giant cell arteritis. *Acta Pathol Microbiol Immunol Scand* 99: 1013–1023

9   Takayasu arteritis and Buerger disease (1998) Report on the IIIrd International Conference on Takayasu arteritis and Buerger disease. *Int J Cardiol* 66 (Suppl 1): S1–290

10 Seko Y (2000) Takayasu arteritis: insights into immunopathology. *Jpn Heart J* 41: 15–26

11 Lhote F, Cohen P, Guillevin L (1998) Polyarteritis nodosa, microscopic polyangiitis and Churg Strauss syndrome. *Lupus* 7: 238–258

12 Watts RA, Jolliffe VA, Carruthers DM, Lockwood M, Scott DG (1996) Effect of classification on the incidence of polyarteritis nodosa and microscopic polyangiitis. *Arthritis Rheum* 39: 1208–1212

13 Guillevin L, Lhote F, Gherardi R (1997) The spectrum and treatment of virus-associated vasculitides. *Curr Opin Rheumatol* 9: 31–36

14 Rowley AH, Shulman ST (1999) Kawasaki syndrome. *Pediatr Clin North Am* 46: 313–329

15 Abe J, Kotzin BL, Jujo K, Melish ME, Glode MP, Kohsaka T, Leung DY (1992) Selective expansion of T cells expressing T-cell receptor variable regions Vβ2 and Vβ8 in Kawasaki disease. *Proc Natl Acad Sci USA* 89: 4066–4070

16 Langford CA, Hoffman GS (1999) Rare diseases 3: Wegener's granulomatosis. *Thorax* 54: 629–637

17 Hoffman GS, Kerr GS, Leavitt RY, Hallahan CW, Lebovics RS, Travis WD (1992) Wegener Granulomatosis: an analysis of 158 patients. *Ann Intern Med* 116: 488–498

18 Laugue D, Cadranel J, Lazor R, Tourrat J, Ronco P, Guillevin L, Cordier JF (2000) Microscopic polyangiitis with alveolar hemorrhage. A study of 29 cases and review of the literature. *Medicine* 79: 222–233

19 Eustace JA, Nadasdy T, Choi M (1999) Disease of the month. The Churg-Strauss syndrome. *J Am Soc Nephrol* 10: 2048–2055

20 Rai A, Nast C, Adler S (1999) Henoch-Schönlein purpura nephritis. *J Am Soc Nephrol* 10: 2637–2644

21 Saulsbury F (1999) Henoch-Schönlein purpura in children. Report of 100 patients and review of the literature. *Medicine* 78: 395–409

22 Lamprecht P, Gause A, Gross WL (1999) Cryoglobulinemic vasculitis. *Arthritis Rheum* 42: 2507–2516

23 McMurray RW (1998) Hepatitis C-associated autoimmune disorders. *Rheum Dis Clin North Am* 24: 353–374

24 Lotti T, Ghersetich I, Comacchi C, Jorizzo JL (1998) Cutaneous small-vessel vasculitis. *J Am Acad Dermatol* 39: 667–687

25   Belizna C, Cohen Tervaert JW (1997) Specificity, pathogenecity, and clinical value of antiendothelial cell antibodies. *Seminars Arthritis Rheum* 27: 98–109

26   Meroni PL, Del Papa N, Raschi E, Tincani A, Balestrieri G, Youinou P (1999) Antiendothelial cell antibodies (AECA): from a laboratory curiosity to another useful autoantibody. In: Y Shoenfeld (ed): *The decade of autoimmunity*. Elsevier Science BV, Amsterdam, 285–294

27   Blank M, Krause I, Goldkorn T et al (1999) Monoclonal anti-endothelial cell antibodies from a patient with Takayasu arteritis activate endothelial cells from large vessels. *Arthritis Rheum* 42: 1421–1432

28   Goldschmeding R, van der Schoot CE, ten Bokkel Huinink D, Hack CE, van den Ende ME, Kallenberg CGM, von dem Borne AEG (1989) Wegener's granulomatosis autoantibodies identify a novel diisopropylfluorophosphate-binding protein in the lysosomes of normal human neutrophils. *J Clin Invest* 84: 1577–1587

29   Hoffman GS, Specks U (1998) Antineutrophil cytoplasmic antibodies. *Arthritis Rheum* 41: 1521–1537

30   Cohen Tervaert JW, van der Woude FJ, Fauci AS, Ambrus JL, Velosa J, Keane WF, Meijer S, van der Giessen M, The TH, van der Hem GK, Kallenberg CGM (1989) Association between active Wegener's granulomatosis and anticytoplasmic antibodies. *Arch Intern Med* 149: 2461–2465

31   Nölle B, Specks V, Lüdemann J, Rohrbach MS, De Remee DA, Gross WL (1989) Anticytoplasmic autoantibodies: their immunodiagnostic value in Wegener's granulomatosis. *Ann Int Med* 111: 28–40

32   Weber MFA, Andrassy K, Pullig O, Koderisch J, Netzer K (1992) Antineutrophil cytoplasmic antibodies and antiglomerular basement membrane antibodies in Goodpasture's syndrome and Wegener's granulomatosis. *J Am Soc Nephrol* 2: 1227–1234

33   Rao JK, Allen NB, Feussner JR, Weinberger M (1995) A prospective study of antineutrophil cytoplasmic antibody (c-ANCA) and clinical criteria in diagnosing Wegener's granulomatosis. *Lancet* 346: 926–931

34   Rao JK, Weinberger M, Oddone EZ, Allen NB, Landsman P, Feussner JR (1995) The role of antineutrophil cytoplasmic antibody testing in the diagnosis of Wegener granulomatosis. *Ann Intern Med* 123: 925–932

35   Cohen Tervaert JW, Goldschmeding R, Elema JD, Limburg PC, Giessen M van der, Huitema MG, Koolen MI, Hené RJ, The TH, Hem GK van der et al (1990) Association of autoantibodies to myeloperoxidase with different forms of vasculitis. *Arthritis Rheum* 33: 1264–1272

36   Cohen Tervaert JW, Limburg PC, Elema JD, Huitema MG, Horst G, The TH, Kallenberg CGM (1991) Detection of autoantibodies against myeloid lysosomal enzymes: a useful adjunct to classification of patients with biopsy-proven necrotizing arteritis. *Am J Med* 91: 59–66

37   Jayne DRW, Marshall PD, Jones SJ, Lockwood CM (1990) Autoantibodies to GBM and neutrophil cytoplasm in rapidly progressive glomerulonephritis. *Kidney Int* 37: 965–970

38   Hagen EC, Daha MR, Hermans J, Andrassy K, Csernok E, Gaskin G, Lesavre P, Lüde-

mann J, Rasmussen N, Sinico RA et al (1998) Diagnostic value of standardized assays for anti-neutrophil cytoplasmic antibodies in idiopathic systemic vasculitis. EC/BCR project for ANCA assay standardization. *Kidney Int* 53: 743–753

39   Cohen Tervaert JW, Huitema MG, Hené RJ, Sluiter WJ, The TH, van der Hem GK, Kallenberg CGM (1990) Prevention of relapses in Wegener's granulomatosis by treatment based on antineutrophil cytoplasmic antibody titre. *Lancet* 336: 709–711

40   Kerr GR, Fleischer THA, Hallahan CD et al (1993) Limited prognostic value of changes in antineutrophil cytoplasmic antibody titer in patients with Wegener's granulomatosis. *Arthritis Rheum* 36: 365–371

41   Boomsma MM, Stegeman CA, van der Leij MJ, Oost W, Herman J, Kallenberg CGM, Limburg PC, Cohen Tervaert JW (2000) Prediction of relapses in Wegener's granulomatosis by measurement of anti neutrophil cytoplasmic antibody levels; a prospective study. *Arthritis Rheum* 43: 2025–2033

42   Stegeman CA, Cohen Tervaert JW, Sluiter WJ, Manson W, Jong PE de, Kallenberg CGM (1994) Association of chronic nasal carriage of *Staphylococcus aureus* and higher relapse rates in Wegener's granulomatosis. *Ann Intern Med* 113: 12–17

43   Falk RJ, Terrell RS, Charles LA, Jennette JC (1990) Anti-neutrophil cytoplasmic autoantibodies induce neutrophils to degranulate and produce oxygen radicals *in vitro*. *Proc Natl Acad Sci USA* 87: 4115–4119

44   Reumaux D, Vossebeld PJ, Roos D, Verhoeven AJ (1995) Effect of tumor necrosis factor-induced integrin activation on Fc gamma receptor II-mediated signal transduction: relevance for activation of neutrophils by anti-proteinase 3 or anti-myeloperoxidase antibodies. *Blood* 86: 3189–3195

45   Brouwer E, Huitema MG, Mulder AHL, Heeringa P, van Goor H, Cohen Tervaert JW, Weening JJ, Kallenberg CGM (1994) Neutrophil activation *in vitro* and *in vivo* in Wegener's granulomatosis. *Kidney Int* 45: 1120–1131

46   Porges AJ, Redecha PB, Kimberly WT, Csernok E, Gross WL, Kimberly RP (1994) Anti-neutrophil cytoplasmic antibodies engage and activate human neutrophils *via* Fc gamma RIIa. *J Immunol* 153: 1271–1278

47   Ewert BH, Jennette JC, Falk RJ (1992) Anti-myeloperoxidase antibodies stimulate neutrophils to damage human endothelial cells. *Kidney Int* 41: 375–383

48   Savage CO, Pottinger BE, Gaskin G, Pusey CD, Pearson JD (1992) Autoantibodies developing to myeloperoxidase and proteinase 3 in systemic vasculitis stimulate neutrophil cytotoxicity toward cultured endothelial cells. *Am J Pathol* 141: 335–342

49   Radford DJ, Savage COS, Nash GB (2000) Treatment of rolling neutrophils with anti-neutrophil cytoplasmic antibodies causes conversion to firm integrin-mediated adhesion. *Arthritis Rheum* 43: 1337–1345

50   Mayet WJ, Csernok E, Szymkowiak C, Gross WL, Meyer zum Büschenfelde KH (1993) Human endothelial cells express proteinase 3, the target antigen of anti-cytoplasmic antibodies in Wegener's granulomatosis. *Blood* 82: 1221–1229

51   Pendergraft WF, Alcorta DA, Segelmark M, Yang JJ, Tuttle R, Jennette JC, Falk RJ, Pre-

ston GA (2000) ANCA antigens, proteinase 3 and myeloperoxidase, are not expressed in endothelial cells. *Kidney Int* 57: 1981–1990

52   Taekema –Roelvink ME, Van Kooten C, Heemskerk E, Schroeijers W, Daha MR (2000) Proteinase 3 interacts with a 111-KD membrane molecule of human umbilical vein endothelial cells. *J Am Soc Nephrol* 11: 640–648

53   Brouwer E, Huitema MG, Klok PA, Cohen Tervaert JW, Weening JJ, Kallenberg CGM (1993) Anti-myeloperoxidase associated proliferative glomerulonephritis: an animal model. *J Exp Med* 177: 905–914

54   Heeringa P, Brouwer E, Klok PA, Huitema MG, Born J van den, Weening JJ, Kallenberg CGM (1996) Autoantibodies to myeloperoxidase aggravate mild anti-glomerular-basement-membrane-mediated glomerular injury in the rat. *Am J Pathol* 149: 1695–1706

55   Heeringa P, Brouwer E, Cohen Tervaert JW, Weening JJ, Kallenberg CGM (1998) Animal models of anti-neutrophil cytoplasmic antibody associated vasculitis. *Kidney Int* 53: 253–263

56   Hunder GG (1998) Giant cell arteritis. *Lupus* 7: 266–269

57   Combe B, Sany J, Le Quellec A, Clot J, Eliaou JF (1998) Distribution of HLA-DRB1 alleles of patients with polymyalgia rheumatica and giant cell arteritis in a Mediterranian population. *J Rheumatol* 25: 94–98

58   Rauzy O, Fort M, Nourhashemi F, Abric L, Juchet H, Ecoiffier M, Abbal M, Adoue M (1999) Relation between HLA DRB1 alleles and corticosteroid resistance in giant cell arteritis. *Ann Rheum Dis* 57: 380–382

59   Martinez-Taboada V, Hunder NN, Hunder GG, Weyand CM, Goronzy JJ (1996) Recognition of tissue residing antigen by T cells in vasculitic lesions of giant cell arteritis. *J Mol Med* 74: 695–703

60   O'Brien JP, Regan W (1998) Actinically degenerated elastic tissue: the prime antigen in the giant cell arteritis syndrome? New data from the posterior ciliary arteries. *Clin Exp Rheumatol* 16: 39–48

61   Brack A, Geisler A, Martinez-Taboada V, Younge BR, Goronzy JJ, Weyand CM (1997) Giant cell arteritis is a T-cell dependent disease. *Mol Med* 3: 530–543

62   Weyand CM, Tetzlaff N, Bjornsson J, Brack A, Younge B, Goronzy JJ (1997) Disease patterns and tissue cytokine profiles in giant cell arteritis. *Arthritis Rheum* 40: 19–26

63   Kaiser M, Weyand CM, Bjornsson J, Goronzy JJ (1998) Platelet-derived growth factor, intimal hyperplasia, and ischemic complications in giant cell arteritis. *Arthritis Rheum* 41: 623–633

64   Weyand CM, Goronzy JJ (1999) Arterial wall injury in giant cell arteritis. *Arthritis Rheum* 42: 844–853

Standard therapeutic regimens for vasculitis

Jan W. Cohen Tervaert[1], Coen A. Stegeman[2] and Cees G.M. Kallenberg[3]

[1]Department of Clinical and Experimental Immunology, University Hospital Maastricht, P.O. Box 5800, 6202 AZ Maastricht, The Netherlands; [2]Department of Internal Medicine, Division of Nephrology, University Hospital Groningen, Hanzeplein 1, 9713 GZ Groningen, The Netherlands; [3]Department of Clinical Immunology, University Hospital Groningen, P.O. Box 30.001, 9700 RB Groningen, The Netherlands

Introduction

Necrotizing systemic vasculitis was described nearly 135 years ago as a fatal condition [1]. Early reports of these forms of vasculitis indeed documented a rapidly progressive course with death occurring within months of diagnosis [2, 3]. Treatment with corticosteroids reduced the 1-year mortality, but after 3 years no difference in mortality was found between treated and untreated patients [4]. Since the introduction of a combination of cyclophosphamide and steroids, however, the outcome of vasculitis has dramatically changed, and 1-year survival has increased to 70–99% [5–9]. Vasculitis has now become a chronic disorder with accumulating morbidity resulting in impairment of employability, functional status, and social activities [10, 11]. The costs for vasculitis-related hospitalizations in the USA were roughly calculated to be over $150 million per year [12]. There is a constant need to improve therapeutic protocols for vasculitis since current protocols are toxic, contribute to morbidity and mortality, and are not always effective. Novel approaches that recently became available include therapy with mycophenolate and/or 15-deoxyspergualin (see the chapter by Stegeman and Birck in this volume), intravenous immunoglobulin (see the chapter by Jayne), tumor necrosis factor α (TNFα) directed therapy (see the chapter by Stone), anti-thymocyte globulin and anti-CD52/anti-CD4 therapy (see the chapter by Schmitt et al.), and immunoablation with or without stem cell rescue (see the chapter by Carruthers and Bacon). These novel approaches offer the possibility to treat patients with a less toxic and/or more effective treatment modality than with the therapeutic regimens that are currently used as "standard regimens". These latter will be reviewed in this chapter.

Disease-modifying Therapy in Vasculitides, edited by Cees G. M. Kallenberg and Jan W. Cohen Tervaert
© 2001 Birkhäuser Verlag Basel/Switzerland

Standard therapy of primary vasculitides

Relatively few randomized-controlled trials have been performed in vasculitis. Much of the evidence supporting therapeutic decisions comes from small prospective or larger retrospective studies. In addition, consensus discussions have set some guidelines for treatment practice.

Vasculitis affecting large-sized blood vessels

Giant cell arteritis/temporal arteritis

In giant cell arteritis/temporal arteritis (GCA) corticosteroids are very effective in suppressing clinical manifestations and immediate relief of symptoms supports the diagnosis of GCA . The purpose of treatment is not only to eliminate pain and other symptoms, but also to prevent blindness and other vascular complications. Recommendations on the initial dose of corticosteroids vary [13]. In an analysis of five prospective studies, Wilke found that symptoms were controlled in 95–97% of GCA patients with an initial dose of prednisone of 11–25 mg/day. Blindness occurred in less than 1 % of the patients. For the small group of patients who present with eye complications and/or severe vascular complications a starting dose of 60 mg/day is recommended [14].

Dose reductions should be started after 1 or 2 weeks under careful monitoring of ESR and CRP. A dose of 15 mg must be reached within 2 months. Thereafter, the prednisone dose may be reduced with 2.5 mg/day every month until a maintenance dose of 5 mg (range, 2.5–7.5 mg) is reached [14]. Maintenance therapy could be stopped if patients are asymptomatic for 6 months on a maintenance dose of 2.5 mg/day. After stopping treatment about 50% of the patients will experience a relapse that can be treated with restarting prednisone at a dose of 10–15 mg/day [14]. Relapses also occur frequently during the first two years after diagnosis when steroids are being tapered off. Weyand et al. [15] used a well-defined tapering protocol, in which patients started on a regimen of 60 mg prednisone daily. The dosage is then tapered according to the following schedule: 10 mg every 2 weeks to 40 mg daily, then 2.5 mg weekly to 20 mg daily, then 2.5 mg every 2 weeks to 10 mg daily, and then 1 mg every month until the patient is no longer being treated. Using this well-defined tapering protocol, they found that only 10 of 25 (40%) patients remained clinically asymptomatic and were able to continue prednisone reductions without any deviation from the protocol [15]. Within a follow-up of 550 days, prednisone could be stopped in 16 patients (64%). Remarkably, IL-6 levels remained elevated in 11 (69%) of these 16 patients despite the absence of clinical disease activity. The high relapse rate and the persistence of elevated IL-6 levels found in this study reinforces the concept that corticosteroids only suppress symptoms but do not eradicate the vasculitic process. Weyand et al. concluded that alternative avenues of treatment warrant exploration [15]. Azathioprine and MTX have been explored as steroid sparing agents. Only small randomized trials have been reported until now (reviewed in [13]). Whereas azathioprine proved to be corticosteroid-sparing in giant cell arteritis/polymyalgia rheumatica [16], 7.5 mg MTX per week was not shown to be significantly corticosteroid-sparing in a double-blind controlled trial in patients with GCA/polymyalgia rheumatica [17]. More recently, Jover et al. [18] reported a randomized, double-blind study in 42 patients with GCA who received corticosteroids, starting dose 60 mg/day followed by a quick-tapering schedule, in combination with either 10 mg MTX per week or placebo during a period of 24 months. During the study, three of 42 patients were lost to follow-up. Relapses occurred more frequently in patients who received placebo (16 of 19 *versus* 9 of 20 in the MTX group; $p = 0.018$). Furthermore, the mean cumulative dose of prednisone was significantly higher in the patients who received placebo (5.490 mg *versus* 4.187 mg in the MTX group; $p = 0.009$). This study demonstrates that MTX is beneficial in GCA. A limiting factor of MTX, however, is its toxicity. Serious MTX-related adverse effects appear to occur in patients not receiving folic acid supplementation or in patients with elevated levels of serum creatinine.

Takayasu arteritis

In Takayasu arteritis (TA) glucocorticosteroids are also the first modality of treatment. Although it has been suggested in older reports that steroids are effective in most patients, it has become clear during the last several years that many patients do not achieve a remission despite high dose (1 mg/kg/day) prednisone and that most of the patients that initially respond will eventually relapse [13]. Since persistence of vascular inflammation in TA may result in severe atherosclerotic complications there is a need to study whether corticosteroids in combination with cytotoxic therapy improve outcome. Randomized trials have not yet been performed in TA. Several cytotoxic drugs such as MTX, azathioprine and cyclophosphamide have been used. A 20-year study from the NIH revealed that 45% of 60 patients had at least one relapse and 23% never achieved a corticosteroid-free remission [19]. In an open-label study in patients with TA, Hoffman et al. reported that MTX induced a remission in 13 of 16 patients, in whom treatment with corticosteroids had previously failed. However, seven of these patients had relapses as corticosteroids were tapered or discontinued [19]. Since cyclophosphamide has relatively more severe short- and long-term side effects than MTX, it is felt that MTX should be preferred in patients with corticosteroid-resistant TA (see the chapter by Langford and Hoffman). In patients with TA special attention must also be paid to risk factors for accelerated atherosclerosis such as hypertension, hypercholesterolaemia, diabetes, and smoking. Hypertension in these patients is often due to renal artery stenosis which can be treated with percutaneous transluminal angioplasty (PTCA) [20].

Vasculitis affecting medium-sized vessels

Kawasaki disease

Kawasaki disease or mucocutaneous lymph node syndrome is a form of systemic vasculitis that mainly affects infants and children under 5 years of age. There is clear ethnic bias towards oriental or Afro-Caribbean children (reviewed in [21]). The principal symptoms include persistent fever, reddening of palms and soles, a polymorphous exanthema, injection of conjunctiva, lips, tongue and/or oral and pharyngeal mucosa, and cervical lymphadenopathy. About 32% of the patients suffer from cardiovascular complications such as coronary artery dilatation, pericarditis and/or cardiac failure. The treatment of choice is low-dose aspirin in combination with high-dose (2 g/kg) intravenous gamma globulin. In patients with severe disease who do not respond to gamma globulin treatment, high-dose steroids are advised [21].

Polyarteritis nodosa

Polyarteritis nodosa (PAN) as recently redefined according to the Chapel Hill Consensus Conference criteria is a form of vasculitis affecting medium-sized and/or small arteries, but not smaller vessels [22]. Consequently, renal failure in PAN is due to vascular nephropathy which may result in (malignant) hypertension. If vasculitis of medium-sized or small arteries is accompanied by glomerulonephritis and/or leukocytoclastic vasculitis of the skin a diagnosis of microscopic polyangiitis (MPA) or one of the other forms of small-vessel vasculitis must be made. PAN is an ANCA negative form of vasculitis and an acute disease in which flares occur in fewer than 10% of the cases [23]. PAN may be attributable to hepatitis B virus infection in less than 10% of the cases [24]. Other well recognized causes of PAN that warrant special attention before choosing the right therapy include other virus infections such as HIV, hepatitis C, and parvovirus B infection, and rare conditions such as hairy cell leukemia and atrial myxoma.

PAN can be treated with corticosteroids as the sole therapy if there is no major organ involvement (i.e., cardiac, gastrointestinal, central nervous, or kidney involvement) [25]. In patients with major organ involvement, cyclophosphamide has to be added [19]. Cyclophosphamide in PAN can be given as IV pulses. Usually doses between 0.5 g–1.5 g are used at intervals between 1–4 weeks. If IV pulse cyclophosphamide fails to induce a remission a switch to oral cyclophosphamide (2.0–2.5 mg/kg/day) is recommended. In case of HBV-related PAN, corticosteroids and immunosuppressive agents may enhance viral replication and may be deleterious. Treatment in HBV-related PAN consists of a short course of corticosteroids, plasma exchange, and anti-viral agents such as lamivudine, interferon α and/or vidarabine [25]. Based on this treatment regimen Guillevin et al. [25] reported a 10-year survival of 83% and a total clearance of HBV in 24% of the cases with HBV-related PAN (see the chapter by Guillevin).

Vasculitis affecting small-sized vessels

ANCA-associated vasculitis and/or glomerulonephritis (AAV)

Patients with Wegener's granulomatosis, Churg-Strauss syndrome, microscopic polyangiitis, and idiopathic necrotizing crescentic glomerulonephritis all belong to the AAV group [26]. It has been questioned whether all patients with AAV need the same strong immunosuppressive treatment. Whereas severe kidney involvement clearly needs to be aggressively treated, it has been known for decades that Wegener's granulomatosis that is limited to the respiratory tract may have an indolent course for years without any form of therapy [27, 28]. During the last decade the European Vasculitis Study Group (EUVAS) proposed a system of clinical subgrouping based on disease severity at presentation. The aim of this subgrouping was to start randomized clinical trials [29, 30]. The following subgroups are recognized: (a) generalized with severe renal involvement, (b) generalized, (c) early systemic, (d) loco-regional, (e) refractory.

Induction of remission

Since induction and maintenance therapy for the different subgroups vary, we will discuss them separately (Tab. 1).

Generalized with severe renal involvement

Patients are treated with daily oral cyclophosphamide (2–3 mg/kg/day) in combination with 1 mg/kg/day prednisone. In addition, when there is severe extrarenal involvement such as alveolar haemorrhage pulsed intravenous methylprednisone (usually three pulses of 1 g) with or without plasma exchange should be added [31]. In patients without severe extrarenal disease there is a potential benefit for the combination of plasma exchange, cyclophosphamide, and corticosteroids [32]. In an analysis of all published data, Levy and Pusey found that 44 of 58 (76%) dialysis-dependent patients who were treated with plasma exchange in combination with conventional treatment came off dialysis, whereas 87 of 151 (58%) patients came off dialysis when treated with corticosteroids and cyclophosphamide only [33].

At present, a prospective study is being performed in which pulses of methylprednisone are being compared with plasma exchange in patients with severe renal involvement ("the MEPEX study") [29].

Generalized disease

Oral cyclophosphamide (2 mg/kg/day) in combination with 1 mg/kg/day prednisone has been the treatment of choice for more than two decades in patients with AAV with generalized disease. Since up to 50% of the patients may experience severe infections that may account for a mortality rate of up to 26% during this form of therapy [34, 35], several studies have been performed in which the cumulative cyclophosphamide dose is reduced by using intravenous pulse therapy [25, 35, 36]. None of these studies was sufficiently powered to make any firm conclusion. In a meta-analysis of these three randomized clinical trials it was concluded that pulse as compared to oral continuous cyclophosphamide is associated with an increased failure to induce remission, with a higher relapse rate, and with less infectious complications and/or leukopenia [37]. The question whether leukopenia and/or infections can be avoided by making adjustments of the oral cyclophosphamide dose long before the nadir of 3.0×10^9 leukocytes/ml is reached, by using lower doses of corticosteroids, and by using co-trimoxazole as PCP prophylaxis is presently being studied in a randomized trial in which intravenous cyclophosphamide is compared with oral continuous cyclophosphamide (CYCLOPS) [30]. MTX can also be used in patients with generalized disease. Langford et al. used MTX 20–25 mg/week in 21 patients with generalized Wegener's granulomatosis [38]. All patients had active glomerulonephritis (serum creatinine levels < 2.5 mg/dl; 220 μmol/l). One of 21 patients died due to an opportunistic infection. The remaining 20 patients all responded well. After a median follow-up of 76 months (range, 20–108), renal function improved in six, was stable in 12, and deteriorated in two patients. These latter two patients were successfully switched to cyclophosphamide [38]. This study suggests that MTX can be used in patients with generalized AAV. Renal function in the patients treated by Langford et al., however, was only mildly impaired (serum creatinine level < 120 μmol/L) in 12 of 21 patients (EUVAS subgroup "early systemic disease"; Tab. 1), whereas the remaining nine patients had mild to moderate renal failure (serum creatinine < 220 μmol/L) (EUVAS subgroup "generalized disease"; Tab. 1).

Since it is at present not clear how safely MTX can be used in patients with more severe renal insufficiency (creatinine clearance < 50 ml/min) an alternative treatment for cyclophosphamide is clearly needed. Recently, it has been proposed that Mycophenolate Mofetil (MMF) can be used in patients with active vasculitis and renal insufficiency [39–43]. We recently treated 13 patients with active Wegener's granulomatosis with MMF (2 g/day) in combination with prednisone (0.5–1.0 mg/kg/day with successive tapering) [42]. All patients were intolerant to cyclophosphamide. All patients responded but relapses occurred in three patients after 5–10 months of follow-up. The other 10 patients came in complete remission during a median follow-up of 14 months (see the chapter by Stegeman and Birck).

Early systemic disease
1.5–2.0 mg/kg/day oral cyclophosphamide in combination with 1 mg/kg/day prednisone has been the standard treatment for early systemic, non-life-threatening disease. While this regimen is often associated with potentially fatal opportunistic

Table 1 - Clinical subgrouping according to disease severity at presentation for ANCA-associated vasculitides

Clinical subgroup	Renal involvement	Serum creatinine (μmol/l)	Standard induction treatment
localized	no	< 120	trimethoprim-sulfamethoxazole
early systemic	yes or no	< 120	cyclophosphamide or MTX + prednisone
generalized	yes	< 500	cyclophosphamide + prednisone
severe renal	yes	> 500	cyclophosphamide + prednisone + plasma exchange or pulse methylprednisone
refractory	yes or no	any	IVIg, anti-CD18, ATG, anti CD52/anti CD4, immunoablation with or without stem cell rescue

IVIg, intravenous immunoglobulin; ATG, antithymocyte globulin

infections (as already stated above) it is felt that patients with non life-threatening disease are "overtreated". Furthermore, cyclophosphamide treatment may be complicated by transitional cell carcinoma of the bladder, and the risk of developing such a cancer may be as high as 16% at 15 years after start of cyclophosphamide treatment [44]. This has led the group of Gross et al. to recommend oral Mesna (natrium-2-mercaptoethanesulfonate) to all patients who are treated with either IV or oral cyclophosphamide [9]. Also the risk of developing other malignancies is increased in patients with AAV that are treated with cyclophosphamide [45].

For these reasons, MTX has been investigated in Wegener's granulomatosis with the hypothesis that it is as effective as cyclophosphamide and less toxic. The results from two open-label studies show remission rates of 70–80% when MTX is used in combination with high-dose corticosteroids [46, 47] and a remission rate of 59% when MTX is combined with lower doses of prednisone (median starting dose of 10 mg/day) [48]. The toxicity of MTX in combination with high-dose corticosteroids was found to be high since 24% of the patients had elevated transaminase levels, 7% had leukopenia, 7% had pneumonitis and 4% of the patients had a fatal PCP pneumonia [46]. Since then, PCP prophylaxis (160 mg trimethoprim/800mg sulfamethoxazole three times weekly) is advocated not only to patients who receive cyclophosphamide but also in those who receive MTX [49]. Whether MTX therapy is complicated by a higher relapse rate than cyclophosphamide treatment has not yet been studied in a prospective randomized study. Such a study has been initiated by the EUVAS (the NORAM study) and will soon be completed [29].

Loco-regional or initial phase disease

Initial phase Wegener's granulomatosis is defined by chronic granulomatous inflammation of the respiratory tract without glomerulonephritis and/or other signs of systemic vasculitis. This form of Wegener's granulomatosis can be treated with trimethoprim-sulfamethoxazole monotherapy (twice 960 mg/day) [50, 51]. A matter of debate is whether patients with arthralgias and elevated levels of C-reactive protein benefit from such a treatment as well. During the last 7 years we treated 20 patients with active loco-regional Wegener's granulomatosis with TS as the only drug. In 17 of 20 patients a remission could be induced. One patient did not respond, and in two patients trimethoprim-sulfamethoxazole had to be stopped due to intolerance. Nine of these 17 patients relapsed after a median follow-up of 14 months, whereas eight patients had a sustained complete remission (unpublished observation). Importantly, nine of our 17 patients in whom a remission could be induced with trimethoprim-sulfamethoxazole monotherapy had elevated CRP levels at diagnosis and five of these suffered from migratory arthralgias, suggesting that patients with loco-regional Wegener's granulomatosis and signs of systemic inflammation can also be treated with this form of treatment.

Maintenance therapy

Seventy to 100% of patients with systemic vasculitis that are treated with cyclophosphamide and high-dose prednisone go into remission.

Prednisone tapering schemes differ widely between centers [29]. To avoid infectious complications during the acute phase of the disease it is generally felt that lowering doses of corticosteroids should be started soon after start of treatment, preferably between 2–6 weeks after diagnosis. Furthermore, there is consensus that prednisone doses should not exceed 5–10 mg/day 3 to 6 months after diagnosis.

Cyclophosphamide tapering: In the original NIH protocol it was recommended that cyclophosphamide is maintained at the starting dose for an additional year after achieving remission [52]. Patients at the NIH came into remission after a median of 12 months [52]. After achieving complete remission cyclophosphamide dose was reduced by 25 mg every 2–3 months. To reduce cyclophosphamide toxicity, we use cyclophosphamide during a much shorter period. We start to reduce the dose of cyclophosphamide already 3 months after diagnosis and stop cyclophosphamide treatment 15–18 months after diagnosis [53].

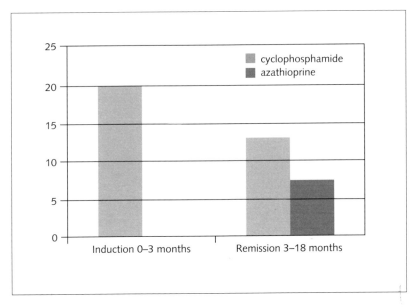

Figure 1

Frequency of severe and life-threatening adverse effects in the CYCAZAREM trial. Patients with ANCA-associated vasculitis were treated with oral cyclophosphamide in combination with prednisone during the induction phase (0–3 months) and subsequently randomized for a maintenance therapy with either cyclophosphamide or azathioprine (3–18 months). From D. Jayne [6], with permission.

Alternative maintenance regimens have been recently proposed to reduce cyclophosphamide exposure. Firstly, a large EUVAS randomized clinical trial comparing azathioprine and continuous cyclophosphamide (CYCAZAREM) have been completed and preliminary results have been reported [6, 30, 54]. One hundred and fifty-five patients entered the study. Following induction of remission with cyclophosphamide and prednisone, 147 patients were randomized to a tapering scheme of oral cyclophosphamide or azathioprine (starting at 150 mg/day) as maintenance therapy. At the end of the study, 18 months after starting therapy, no differences were found in relapse rate between both limbs. There was a trend, however, that serious adverse effects occurred less frequently in the azathioprine limb (Fig. 1).

Cyclophosphamide for induction and MTX as maintenance therapy once remission has been reached is another regimen that has been recently tested in patients with Wegener's granulomatosis. De Groot et al. reported that remission could be maintained in 19 of 22 patients who received MTX as monotherapy (median follow-up: 16 months), whereas remission could be maintained in 10 of 11 patients who received MTX in combination with low-dose prednisone (median follow-up: 22 months) [55]. In another open label trial, Langford et al. tested 20–25 mg/week MTX as maintenance therapy in 31 patients; in 84% of those patients remission could be maintained (median follow-up 16 months) [49]. Cyclosporin and/or MMF have also been tested in small studies as maintenance therapy. No relapses were observed in seven patients with AAV during low-dose cyclosporin (blood levels 60–90 ng/ml) in combination with low-dose prednisone (median follow-up after cyclophosphamide discontinuation: 22 months) [56]. Finally, MMF in combination with low-dose steroids has been used as maintenance therapy in 11 patients with AAV after remission was induced with cyclophosphamide [57]. During a follow-up of 15 months one of these 11 patients suffered from a relapse [57]. In summary, recent studies with either azathioprine, MTX, cyclosporin, or MMF indicate that long-term use of cyclophosphamide can be avoided by using one of these drugs after a remission is induced with cyclophosphamide in combination with high-dose steroids.

Another strategy in AAV patients could be to stop all immunosuppressive drugs 12–18 months after diagnosis [53] and to treat only patients who are identified as "high risk" patients. During the last decade our group studied such a targeted preventive approach [58–62]. In a randomized clinical trial we found that treatment with trimethoprim-sulfamethoxazole (960 mg b.i.d) for 24 months resulted in maintenance of remission in 82% of patients whereas in only 60% of patients who received placebo a remission was maintained [61]. A drawback of trimethoprim-sulfamethoxazole treatment is that about 20% of patients cannot tolerate the drug. Furthermore, from this study it can be calculated that five patients (95% confidence interval, three to 31 patients) have to be treated for 24 months to prevent one relapse. So, trimethoprim-sulfamethoxazole maintenance therapy should be reserved for those patients who are at high risk to develop relapses (see the chapter by Boomsma et al.).

Refractory cases

IVIg 2g/kg infused over 4 to 5 days is the therapy of choice for Kawasaki's disease and has been used successfully in resistant cases of AAV and other forms of small-vessel vasculitis. Jayne et al. used IVIg as an additional agent to standard immunosuppressive therapy in 26 patients with persistently active AAV; 50% went into complete remission and the remainder into partial remission [63]. Recently, Jayne et al. [64] reported the results of a randomized, placebo-controlled trial in 34 patients patients with AAV who suffered from persistently active vasculitis despite standard immunosuppressive treatment. A single course of IVIg induced more frequently a 50% reduction of disease activity in patients who were treated with IVIg (14/17) than in those treated with placebo infusions (6/17). After 3 months, however, no difference was found in the occurrence of relapses: 5/16 patients treated with IVIg relapsed and 4/15 treated with placebo. During IVIg therapy adverse effects were relatively frequently observed: 4/17 patients had reversible rises in serum creatinine and one patient had aseptic meningitis. This study confirms earlier reports that IVIg is effective in AAV. Its effect, however, seems to be relatively weak (see the chapter by Jayne).

For progressive disease resistant to standard therapy or where standard therapy is not tolerated lymphocyte depletion using antithymocyte globulin (ATG) or monoclonal anti-T cell antibodies has induced remissions in small series of patients [65–68]. Recently, Van der Woude et al. reported that ATG induced a complete remission in one of 10 patients with refractory Wegener's granulomatosis, a partial remission in eight of 10 patients, and one patient died due to active disease [68]. Lockwood et al. treated 17 patients with refractory Wegener's granulomatosis with monoclonal antibodies to CD52 followed by a non-depleting antibody to CD4 in courses lasting 5 days each [69]. The anti CD 52 antibody is lytic for all lymphocytes except for natural killer cells. Remission was induced in 16 of 17 patients. During follow-up cytotoxic drugs could be stopped in responders. In 9 of 16 patients, however, relapses occurred. Despite long periods of CD4 depletion in all patients none of the patients suffered from complications such as opportunistic infections or lymphomas [69] (see the chapter by Schmitt et al.).

Another attractive approach for treatment of refractory cases is the use of drugs that inhibit adhesion of leukocytes to endothelial cells (reviewed in [70]). Lockwood et al. [71] recently reported the use of a humanized monoclonal anti-CD18 antibody, genetically engineered to abrogate Fc interactions, in five patients with vasculitic tissue injury that resulted in ulceration and/or limb/digital infarction with incipient gangrene. Remarkable prompt clinical healing of ulceration and restoration of limb function was noted in four of five patients [71]. Finally, immunoablation using high-dose cytotoxic medication with or without stem cell rescue has led to prolonged remission in a few patients with refractory vasculitis [72] (see the chapter by Carruthers and Bacon).

Henoch-Schonlein purpura (HSP)

HSP is usually a self-limited disease with a good clinical outcome [73]. The average duration of a HSP attack is 1 month. Joint pain is effectively treated with non-steroidal anti-inflammatory agents. In addition, corticosteroids may accelerate the resolution of arthritis and abdominal pain. Severe and/or recurrent skin lesions may be treated with oral corticosteroids or 50–100 mg/day dapsone (= diaphenyl-sulphone) [73–75]. In patients with renal disease a renal biopsy is useful for assessing prognosis and suggesting the need for treatment [73]. The treatment of HSP nephritis is controversial and recommendations are mostly based on small uncontrolled series. Since severe crescentic HSP nephritis may progress to end-stage renal failure, treatment of these patients is warranted. Niaudet et al. [76] treated 32 patients with severe HSP nephritis with methylprednisone pulse therapy followed by oral prednisone. Despite this treatment 13% progressed to ESRD and 13% had chronic renal failure [76]. Somewhat better results can probably be obtained by using a combination of cyclophosphamide and/or azathioprine and prednisone (reviewed in [73]). Interestingly, Hattori et al. used plasma exchange as the sole therapy of crescentic HSP nephritis in nine patients. They found a prompt improvement of renal function and proteinuria in combination with disappearance of purpura and abdominal pain in all patients. After stopping plasma exchange, three of nine patients showed a rebound of proteinuria that was accompanied by progression to ESRD in two [77].

Mixed essential cryoglobulinaemia (MEC)

MEC with type II cryoglobulins (polyclonal IgG and monoclonal IgM rheumatoid factor) is secondary to hepatitis C infection in the large majority of patients. The protocols designed for treatment of uncomplicated HCV infection, however, are inadequate for treating MEC secondary to HCV [78]. The end point of treatment of the latter should be complete clearance of both HCV and cryoglobulins. Since standard IFNα therapy (3 × 3 million U/week) is often unsuccessful, daily high doses are recommended [79]. Another approach that was recently reported by Zuckerman et al. [80] was treatment with a combination therapy of IFNα (3 × 3 million U/week) and ribavirin (1000–1200 mg/day; dose adjusted to 400–600 mg/day in patients with impaired renal function). Nine patients were treated and all showed clinical improvement in combination with disappearance of cryoglobulin (seven patients) or decrease in cryoglobulins (two patients). Complete and sustained virological (negative HCV-RNA) remission after 6 months of therapy was, however, observed in two patients only [80]. Calleja et al. [81] recently reported outcome of therapy in 18 patients with MEC due to HCV. Only five of 18 patients demonstrated a sustained response to standard IFNα therapy. During combined IFNα + ribavirin treatment seven of the 13 remaining patients had a sustained response [81]. Continuous administration of IFNα with pegylated IFNα is another available option [78].

In patients with severe vasculitic symptoms such as leg ulcers plasma exchange or cryofiltration with a cooling unit [82] is indicated. In addition, low-dose steroids are sometimes needed, although corticosteroids and immunosuppressives are relatively contraindicated because they may worsen HCV viraemia.

When cryoglobulinaemia develops in a patient without hepatitis C infection but in association with a specific myeloproliferative disorder, then treatment must be directed at the underlying disorder. If neither HCV infection nor a myeloproliferative disorder is present corticosteroids are useful for extrarenal symptoms. When glomerulonephritis is present the traditional approach is corticosteroids, cyclophosphamide and plasma exchange [83].

Idiopathic leukocytoclastic angiitis

Most patients have only minimal or moderate discomfort and no systemic therapy is required. In patients with severe skin lesions corticosteroids may be needed. In chronic cases, dapsone, thalidomide, antimalarials, colchicine, pentoxyfillin, and/or antihistamines may be tried [84]. Only occasionally azathioprine is indicated.

Adverse effects

Adverse effects of treatment are an extremely important contributor to morbidity and mortality in patients with vasculitis. Both immediate and late toxicity is significant. Hoffman et al. reported that treatment toxicity contributed to permanent damage in more than 50% of their patients with Wegener's granulomatosis [52]. More recently, Jayne [6] reported that patients with either Wegener's granulomatosis or microscopic polyangiitis who participated in the CYCAZAREM trial experienced an adverse effect frequency of 1.1 episodes per patient within the first 18 months after diagnosis. In 26% of the patients side-effects were severe or life-threatening. Infectious adverse effects are the most common cause of death or severe morbidity. Their frequency is increased in patients of older age and is related to steroid doses. Patients are at increased risk of cytomegalovirus, aspergillus, candida, herpes zoster and pneumocystis carinii infection. In addition, nocardia and reactivation of tuberculosis may occur. Bacteria infections, especially due to staphylococcus aureus, are also frequently observed and may be severe. Routine prophylaxis with oral amphotericin B and low-dose sulphamethoxazole/trimethoprim is warranted. The role of prophylactic acyclovir and/or ganciclovir is not clear in patients with vasculitis. In patients with a history of tuberculosis prophylactic isoniazide may be considered. Late toxicities due to cyclophosphamide include haemorrhagic cystitis, bladder fibrosis and/or bladder carcinoma. To limit this toxicity, cyclophosphamide should be given in the morning and combined with a high fluid intake if renal function allows such a policy. In addition, mesna should be administrated either intravenously or orally [9] when high-dose pulsed cyclophosphamide is used or when the cumulative dose of oral cyclophosphamide is expected to become more than 100 g [44]. Whether patients with a short course of oral cyclophosphamide have also an increased risk of bladder carcinoma and should also receive mesna remains to be investigated. Immunosuppressive therapy also increases the risk of other malignancies [45]. Especially the risk of skin cancer is increased and it seems prudent to advise all patients to reduce sun exposure. Other important toxicities include infertility, steroid-induced osteoporosis, and accelerated atherosclerosis. Osteoporosis prophylaxis should include calcium supplementation and activated vitamin D. In addition, hormone replacement therapy may be considered in post-menopausal females. Finally, biphosphonates may be used in patients with an established decrease in bone mineral density (renal function permitting). Accelerated athero-sclerosis did not receive much attention yet in patients with vasculitis. Accelerated atherosclerosis is not only due to persistent activity of vasculitis, but also to chron-ic treatment with steroids resulting in increased levels of cholesterol, higher blood pressure levels and weight gain [85]. Since no randomized trials have been conduct-ed that prove that aggressive anti-atherosclerotic regimens with cholesterol lower-ing drugs and ACE inhibitors are beneficial in patients with vasculitis, the European Vasculitis Study Group is currently planning such trials.

Conclusions

High-dose corticosteroids with or without cytotoxic drugs such as cyclophos-phamide and methotrexate are used to induce a remission in giant cell arteritis, Takayasu arteritis, PAN and the ANCA-associated vasculitides. If cyclophos-phamide is used for induction therapy it is recommended to use either azathioprine or methotrexate for maintenance therapy. For Kawasaki disease IVIg in combina-tion with acetylsalicylic acid is the first treatment option, whereas in hepatitis B and/or C associated vasculitis IFNα in combination with other antiviral drugs must be used. Finally, for loco-regional Wegener's granulomatosis trimethoprim-sul-famethoxazole monotherapy can be used, whereas for vasculitis localized to the skin dapsone monotherapy is often sufficiently effective. The current studies in which newer immunosuppressives are being tested offer exciting new possibilities for treat-ment of vasculitis patients. Many of these new approaches will be discussed in the next chapters.

References

1   Kussmaul A, Maier K (1866) Ueber eine bisher nicht beschriebene eigentümliche Arte-rienkrankung (Periarteriitis Nodosa), die mit morbus Brightii und rapid fortschreitender allgemeiner Muskellähmung einhergeht. *Deutsch Arch f Klin Med* 1: 484–517

2   Walton EW (1958) Giant cell granuloma of the respiratory tract (Wegener's granulo-matosis). *BMJ* 2: 265–270

3   Frohnert PP, Sheps SG (1967) Long-term follow-up study of periarteritis nodosa. *Am J Med* 43: 8–14

4   (1960) Treatment of polyarteritis nodosa with cortisone: results after three years. *BMJ* 4: 1399–1400

5   Gaskin G, Pusey CD (1999) Crescentic glomerulonephritis and systemic vasculitis. In: CD Pusey (ed): *The treatment of glomerulonephritis*. Kluwer Academic Publishers, Dor-drecht, 113–142

6   Jayne D (2000) Evidence-based treatment of systemic vasculitis. *Rheumatology* 39: 585–595

7   McLaughlin K, Jerimiah P, Fox JG, Mactier RA, Simpson K, Boulton-Jones JM (1998) Has the prognosis for patients with pauci-immune necrotizing glomerulonephritis improved? *Nephrol Dial Transplant* 13: 1696–1701

8   Aasarod K, Iversen BM, Hammerstrom J, Bostad L, Vatten L, Jorstad S (2000) Wegener's granulomatosis: clinical course in 108 patients with renal involvement. *Nephrol Dial Transplant* 15: 611–618

9   Reinhold-Keller E, Beuge N, Latza U, de Groot K, Rudert H, Nolle B, Heller M, Gross WL (2000) An interdisciplinary approach to the care of patients with Wegener's granulomatosis: long-term outcome in 155 patients. *Arthritis Rheum* 43: 1021–1032

10   Hoffman GS, Drucker Y, Cotch MF, Locker GA, Easley K, Kwoh K (1998) Wegener's granulomatosis: patient-reported effects of disease on health, function, and income. *Arthritis Rheum* 41: 2257–2262

11   Boomsma MM, Stegeman CA, Cohen Tervaert JW (1999) Comparison of Dutch and US patients' perceptions of the effects of Wegener's granulomatosis on health, function, income, and interpersonal relationships: comment on the article by Hoffman et al. [letter]. *Arthritis Rheum* 42: 2495–2497

12   Cotch MF (2000) The socioeconomic impact of vasculitis. *Curr Opin Rheumatol* 12: 20–23

13   Wilke WS (1997) Large vessel vasculitis (giant cell arteritis, Takayasu arteritis). *Baillieres Clin Rheumatol* 11: 285–313

14   Nordborg E, Nordborg C, Malmvall BE, Andersson R, Bengtsson BA (1995) Giant cell arteritis. *Rheum Dis Clin North Am* 21: 1013–1026

15   Weyand CM, Fulbright JW, Hunder GG, Evans JM, Goronzy JJ (2000) Treatment of giant cell arteritis: interleukin-6 as a biologic marker of disease activity. *Arthritis Rheum* 43: 1041–1048

16   De Silva M, Hazleman BL (1986) Azathioprine in giant cell arteritis/polymyalgia rheumatica: a double-blind study. *Ann Rheum Dis* 45: 136–138

17   Van der Veen MJ, Dinant HJ, Van Booma-Frankfort C, Van Albada–Kuipers GA, Bijlsma JW (1996) Can methotrexate be used as a steroid sparing agent in the treatment of polymyalgia rheumatica and giant cell arteritis? *Ann Rheum Dis* 55: 218–223

18   Jover J, Hernández-García C, Morado I, Vargas E, Bañares A, Fernández-Gutiérrez B (2001) Combined treatment of giant cell arteritis with methotrexate and prednisone: a randomized, double blind, and placebo-controlled study. *Ann Intern Med* 134: 106–114

19   Hoffman GS, Leavitt RY, Kerr GS, Rottem M, Sneller MC, Fauci AS (1994) Treatment of glucocorticoid-resistant or relapsing Takayasu arteritis with methotrexate. *Arthritis Rheum* 37: 578–582

20   Tyagi S, Singh B, Kaul UA, Sethi KK, Arora R, Khalilullah M (1993) Balloon angioplasty for renovascular hypertension in Takayasu's arteritis. *Am Heart J* 125: 1386–1393

21   Dillon MJ, Ansell BM (1995) Vasculitis in children and adolescents. *Rheum Dis Clin North Am* 21: 1115–1136

22   Jennette JC, Falk RJ, Andrassy K, Bacon PA, Churg J, Gross WL, Hagen EC, Hoffman GS, Hunder GG, Kallenberg CG et al (1994) Nomenclature of systemic vasculitides. Proposal of an international consensus conference. *Arthritis Rheum* 37: 187–192

23   Guillevin L (1999) Treatment of classic polyarteritis nodosa in 1999 [editorial]. *Nephrol Dial Transplant* 14: 2077–2079

24   Lhote F, Guillevin L (1995) Polyarteritis nodosa, microscopic polyangiitis, and Churg-Strauss syndrome. Clinical aspects and treatment. *Rheum Dis Clin North Am* 21: 911–947

25   Guillevin L, Lhote F (1998) Treatment of polyarteritis nodosa and microscopic polyangiitis. *Arthritis Rheum* 41: 2100–2105

26   Franssen CF, Stegeman CA, Kallenberg CG, Gans RO, De Jong PE, Hoorntje SJ, Tervaert JW (2000) Antiproteinase 3- and antimyeloperoxidase-associated vasculitis. *Kidney Int* 57: 2195–2206

27   Fienberg R (1981) The protacted superficial phenomenon in pathergic (Wegener's) granulomatosis. *Hum Path* 12: 458–467

28   Cohen Tervaert JW, van der Woude FJ, Kallenberg CG (1987) Analysis of symptoms preceding the diagnosis of Wegener's disease. *Ned Tijdschr Geneeskd* 131: 1391–1394

29   Rasmussen NJ, Abramowicz D, Andrassy K et al (1995) European therapeutic trials in ANCA-associated systemic vasculitis: disease scoring, consensus regimens and proposed clinical trials. *Clin Exp Immunol* 101 (Suppl 1): 29–34

30   Jayne D, Rasmussen N (2000) European collaborative trials in vasculitis: EUVAS update and latest results. *Clin Exp Immunol* 120 (Suppl 1): 13–15

31   Klemmer PJ, Chalermskulrat W, Reif MS, Hogan SL, Henke DC, Falk RJ (2000) Treatment with plasmapheresis in diffuse alveolar hemorrhage in ANCA-SVV [abstract]. *Clin Exp Immunol* 120 (Suppl 1): 73

32   Pusey CD, Rees AJ, Evans DJ, Peters DK, Lockwood CM (1991) Plasma exchange in focal necrotizing glomerulonephritis without anti-GBM antibodies. *Kidney Int* 40: 757–763

33   Levy JB, Pusey CD (1997) Still a role for plasma exchange in rapidly progressive glomerulonephritis? *J Nephrol* 10: 7–13

34   Guillevin L, Cordier JF, Lhote F, Cohen P, Jarrousse B, Royer I, Lesavre P, Jacquot C, Bindi P, Bielefeld P, et al. (1997) A prospective, multicenter, randomized trial comparing steroids and pulse cyclophosphamide versus steroids and oral cyclophosphamide in the treatment of generalized Wegener's granulomatosis. *Arthritis Rheum* 40: 2187–2198

35   Haubitz M, Schellong S, Gobel U, Schurek HJ, Schaumann D, Koch KM, Brunkhorst R (1998) Intravenous pulse administration of cyclophosphamide versus daily oral treatment in patients with antineutrophil cytoplasmic antibody-associated vasculitis and renal involvement: a prospective, randomized study. *Arthritis Rheum* 41: 1835–1844

36   Adu D, Pall A, Luqmani RA, Richards NT, Howie AJ, Emery P, Michael J, Savage CO,

Bacon PA (1997) Controlled trial of pulse versus continuous prednisolone and cyclophosphamide in the treatment of systemic vasculitis. *QJM* 90: 401–409

37 de Groot K, Adu D, Savage CO (2000) To pulse or not to pulse in ANCA-associated vasculitis – a critical analysis [abstract]. *Clin Exp Immunol* 120 (Suppl 1): 68

38 Langford CA, Talar-Williams C, Sneller MC (2000) Use of methotrexate and glucocorticoids in the treatment of Wegener's granulomatosis. Long-term renal outcome in patients with glomerulonephritis. *Arthritis Rheum* 43: 1836–1840

39 Haidinger M, Neumann L, Jaeger H, Gruetzmacher H, Bayer P, Meisl FT (2000) Mycophenolate Mofetil (MMF) treatment of ANCA-associated small-vessel vasculitis [abstract]. *Clin Exp Immunol* 120 (Suppl 1): 72

40 Nachman PH, Joy MS, Hogan SL, Jennette JC, Falk RJ (2000) Mycophenolate mofetil: preliminary results of a feasibility trial in relapsing ANCA small vessel vasculitis [abstract]. *Clin Exp Immunol* 120 (Suppl 1): 72

41 Pasavento RE, Falkenhain ME, Rovin BH, Hebert LA (1999) Mycophenolate in anti-neutrophil cytoplasmic antibody vasculitis [abstract]. *J Am Soc Nephrol* 10: 114A

42 Stegeman CA, Cohen Tervaert JW (2000) Mycophenolate mofetil for remission induction in patients with active Wegener's granulomatosis intolerant to cyclophosphamide [abstract]. *J Am Soc Nephrol* 11: 98A

43 Waiser J, Budde K, Braasch E, Neumayer HH (1999) Treatment of acute c-ANCA-positive vasculitis with mycophenolate mofetil. *Am J Kidney Dis* 34: e9

44 Talar-Williams C, Hijazi YM, Walther MM, Linehan WM, Hallahan CW, Lubensky I, Kerr GS, Hoffman GS, Fauci AS, Sneller MC (1996) Cyclophosphamide-induced cystitis and bladder cancer in patients with Wegener granulomatosis. *Ann Intern Med* 124: 477–484

45 Westman KW, Bygren PG, Olsson H, Ranstam J, Wieslander J (1998) Relapse rate, renal survival, and cancer morbidity in patients with Wegener's granulomatosis or microscopic polyangiitis with renal involvement. *J Am Soc Nephrol* 9: 842–852

46 Sneller MC, Hoffman GS, Talar-Williams C, Kerr GS, Hallahan CW, Fauci AS (1995) An analysis of forty-two Wegener's granulomatosis patients treated with methotrexate and prednisone. *Arthritis Rheum* 38: 608–613

47 Stone JH, Tun W, Hellman DB (1999) Treatment of non-life threatening Wegener's granulomatosis with methotrexate and daily prednisone as the initial therapy of choice. *J Rheumatol* 26: 1134–1139

48 de Groot K, Muhler M, Reinhold-Keller E, Paulsen J, Gross WL (1998) Induction of remission in Wegener's granulomatosis with low dose methotrexate. *J Rheumatol* 25: 492–495

49 Langford CA, Talar-Williams C, Barron KS, Sneller MC (1999) A staged approach to the treatment of Wegener's granulomatosis: induction of remission with glucocorticoids and daily cyclophosphamide switching to methotrexate for remission maintenance. *Arthritis Rheum* 42: 2666–2673

50 Reinhold-Keller E, De Groot K, Rudert H, Nolle B, Heller M, Gross WL (1996) Response to trimethoprim/sulfamethoxazole in Wegener's granulomatosis depends on

the phase of disease. *QJM* 89: 15–23

51 Stegeman CA, Cohen Tervaert JW, Kallenberg CG (1997) Co-trimoxazole and Wegener's granulomatosis: more than a coincidence? [editorial]. *Nephrol Dial Transplant* 12: 652–655

52 Hoffman GS, Kerr GS, Leavitt RY, Hallahan CW, Lebovics RS, Travis WD, Rottem M, Fauci AS (1992) Wegener granulomatosis: an analysis of 158 patients. *Ann Intern Med* 116: 488–498

53 Franssen CF, Stegeman CA, Oost-Kort WW, Kallenberg CG, Limburg PC, Tiebosch A, De Jong PE, Cohen Tervaert JW (1998) Determinants of renal outcome in anti-myeloperoxidase-associated necrotizing crescentic glomerulonephritis. *J Am Soc Nephrol* 9: 1915–1923

54 Jayne D, Gaskin G (1999) Randomised trial of cyclophosphamide versus azthioprine during remission in ANCA-associated vasculitis (CYCAZAREM) [abstract]. *J Am Soc Nephrol* 10: 105A

55 de Groot K, Reinhold-Keller E, Tatsis E, Paulsen J, Heller M, Nolle B, Gross WL (1996) Therapy for the maintenance of remission in sixty-five patients with generalized Wegener's granulomatosis. Methotrexate versus trimethoprim/sulfamethoxazole. *Arthritis Rheum* 39: 2052–2061

56 Haubitz M, Koch KM, Brunkhorst R (1998) Cyclosporin for the prevention of disease reactivation in relapsing ANCA-associated vasculitis. *Nephrol Dial Transplant* 13: 2074–2076

57 Nowack R, Gobel U, Klooker P, Hergesell O, Andrassy K, van der Woude FJ (1999) Mycophenolate mofetil for maintenance therapy of Wegener's granulomatosis and microscopic polyangiitis: a pilot study in 11 patients with renal involvement. *J Am Soc Nephrol* 10: 1965–1971

58 Cohen Tervaert JW, van der Woude FJ, Fauci AS, Ambrus JL, Velosa J, Keane WF, Meijer S, van der Giessen M, van der Hem GK, The TH et al (1989) Association between active Wegener's granulomatosis and anticytoplasmic antibodies. *Arch Intern Med* 149: 2461–2465

59 Cohen Tervaert JW, Huitema MG, Hene RJ, Sluiter WJ, The TH, van der Hem GK, Kallenberg CG (1990) Prevention of relapses in Wegener's granulomatosis by treatment based on antineutrophil cytoplasmic antibody titre. *Lancet* 336: 709–711

60 Stegeman CA, Cohen Tervaert JW, Sluiter WJ, Manson WL, de Jong PE, Kallenberg CG (1994) Association of chronic nasal carriage of *Staphylococcus aureus* and higher relapse rates in Wegener granulomatosis. *Ann Intern Med* 120: 12–17

61 Stegeman CA, Cohen Tervaert JW, de Jong PE, Kallenberg CG (1996) Trimethoprim-sulfamethoxazole (co-trimoxazole) for the prevention of relapses of Wegener's granulomatosis. Dutch Co-Trimoxazole Wegener Study Group. *N Engl J Med* 335: 16–20

62 Boomsma MM, Stegeman CA, van der Leij MJ, Oost W, Hermans J, Kallenberg CG, Limburg PC, Cohen Tervaert JW (2000) Prediction of relapses in Wegener's granulomatosis by measurement of antineutrophil cytoplasmic antibody levels: a prospective study. *Arthritis Rheum* 43: 2025–2033

63   Jayne DR, Davies MJ, Fox CJ, Black CM, Lockwood CM (1991) Treatment of systemic vasculitis with pooled intravenous immunoglobulin. *Lancet* 337: 1137–1139

64   Jayne DR, Chapel H, Adu D, Misbah S, O'Donoghue D, Scott D, Lockwood CM (2000) Intravenous immunoglobulin for ANCA-associated systemic vasculitis with persistent disease activity. *QJM* 93: 433–439

65   Kjellstrand CM, Simmons RL, Uranga VM, Buselmeier TJ, Najarian JS (1974) Acute fulminant Wegener granulomatosis. Therapy with immunosuppression, hemodialysis, and renal transplantation. *Arch Intern Med* 134: 40–43

66   Hagen EC, de Keizer RJ, Andrassy K, van Boven WP, Bruijn JA, van Es LA, van der Woude FJ (1995) Compassionate treatment of Wegener's granulomatosis with rabbit anti- thymocyte globulin. *Clin Nephrol* 43: 351–359

67   Lockwood CM, Thiru S, Isaacs JD, Hale G, Waldmann H (1993) Long-term remission of intractable systemic vasculitis with monoclonal antibody therapy. *Lancet* 341: 1620–1622

68   Van der Woude FJ, Schmitt WH, Birck R, Nowack R, Gobel U, Drexler JM, Hotta O (2000) New immodulating concepts in ANCA-associated disease. *Clin Exp Immunol* 120 (Suppl 1): 16

69   Lockwood CM (1998) Refractory Wegener's granulomatosis: a model for shorter immunotherapy of autoimmune diseases. *JR Coll Physicians Lond* 32: 473–478

70   Cohen Tervaert JW, Kallenberg CG (2000) Leukocyte cell adhesion molecules in vasculitis. In: R Asherson, R Cervers, D Tripplet, S Abramson (eds): *Vascular manifestations of systemic autoimmune diseases*. CRC Press, London, 161–178

71   Lockwood CM, Elliott JD, Brettman L, Hale G, Rebello P, Frewin M, Ringler D, Merrill C, Waldmann H (1999) Anti-adhesion molecule therapy as an interventional strategy for autoimmune inflammation. *Clin Immunol* 93: 93–106

72   Tyndall A, Fassas A, Passweg J, Ruiz de Elvira C, Attal M, Brooks P, Black C, Durez P, Finke J, Forman S et al (1999) Autologous haematopoietic stem cell transplants for autoimmune disease – feasibility and transplant-related mortality. Autoimmune Disease and Lymphoma Working Parties of the European Group for Blood and Marrow Transplantation, the European League Against Rheumatism and the International Stem Cell Project for Autoimmune Disease. *Bone Marrow Transplant* 24: 729–734

73   Rai A, Nast C, Adler S (1999) Henoch-Schonlein purpura nephritis. *J Am Soc Nephrol* 10: 2637–2644

74   Hoffbrand BI (1991) Dapsone in Henoch-Schonlein purpura – worth a trial [editorial]. *Postgrad Med J* 67: 961–962

75   Albrecht J, Mempel M, Hein R, Abeck D, Ring J (1999) Henoch-Schonlein purpura: successful treatment with Dapsone. *Hautarzt* 50: 809–811

76   Niaudet P, Habib R (1998) Methylprednisolone pulse therapy in the treatment of severe forms of Schonlein-Henoch purpura nephritis. *Pediatr Nephrol* 12: 238–243

77   Hattori M, Ito K, Konomoto T, Kawaguchi H, Yoshioka T, Khono M (1999) Plasmapheresis as the sole therapy for rapidly progressive Henoch- Schonlein purpura nephritis in children. *Am J Kidney Dis* 33: 427–433

78 Agnello V (2000) Therapy for cryoglobulinemia secondary to hepatitis C virus: the need for tailored protocols and multiclinic studies [editorial]. *J Rheumatol* 27: 2065–2067

79 Casato M, Agnello V, Pucillo LP, Knight GB, Leoni M, Del Vecchio S, Mazzilli C, Antonelli G, Bonomo L (1997) Predictors of long-term response to high-dose interferon therapy in type II cryoglobulinemia associated with hepatitis C virus infection. *Blood* 90: 3865–3873

80 Zuckerman E, Keren D, Slobodin G, Rosner I, Rozenbaum M, Toubi E, Sabo E, Tsykounov I, Naschitz JE, Yeshurun D (2000) Treatment of refractory, symptomatic, hepatitis C virus related mixed cryoglobulinemia with ribavirin and interferon-alpha. *J Rheumatol* 27: 2172–2178

81 Calleja JL, Albillos A, Moreno-Otero R, Rossi I, Cacho G, Domper F, Yebra M, Escartin P (1999) Sustained response to interferon-alpha or to interferon-alpha plus ribavirin in hepatitis C virus-associated symptomatic mixed cryoglobulinaemia. *Aliment Pharmacol Ther* 13: 1179–1186

82 Kiyomoto H, Hitomi H, Hosotani Y, Hashimoto M, Uchida K, Kurokouchi K, Nagai M, Takahashi N, Fukunaga M, Mizushige K et al (1999) The effect of combination therapy with interferon and cryofiltration on mesangial proliferative glomerulonephritis originating from mixed cryoglobulinemia in chronic hepatitis C virus infection. *Ther Apher* 3: 329–333

83 Houwert DA, Hene RJ, Struyvenberg A, Kater L (1980) Effect of plasmapheresis (PP), corticosteroids and cyclophosphamide in essential mixed polyclonal cryoglobulinaemia associated with glomerulonephritis. *Proc Eur Dial Transplant Assoc* 17: 650–654

84 Mat C, Yurdakul S, Tuzuner N, Tuzun Y (1997) Small vessel vasculitis and vasculitis confined to skin. *Baillieres Clin Rheumatol* 11: 237–257

85 Petri M, Lakatta C, Magder L, Goldman D (1994) Effect of prednisone and hydroxychloroquine on coronary artery disease risk factors in systemic lupus erythematosus: a longitudinal data analysis. *Am J Med* 96: 254–259

Tumor necrosis factor (TNF) inhibition in the treatment of vasculitis

John H. Stone

The Johns Hopkins Vasculitis Center, 1830 E. Monument Street, Suite 7500, Baltimore, MD 21205, USA

Introduction

Insight into the central roles of cytokines in many inflammatory disorders represents one of the major medical advances of the 1990s. During the last decade, molecular biology provided not only the techniques to investigate individual cytokines in inflammation, but also successful strategies for the inhibition of these cytokines. As described below, the identification of tumor necrosis factor (TNF) as a critical cytokine in the pathophysiology of rheumatoid arthritis (RA) and Crohn's disease has revolutionized the treatment of these diseases [1–10]. The extrapolation and rigorous testing of cytokine modulation strategies in the vasculitides have enormous potential to improve therapies for this group of disorders.

In this chapter, the biologic functions of TNF, the use of anti-TNF therapies in specific inflammatory conditions, the putative role of TNF in the pathophysiology of vasculitis, and current plans to investigate the role of TNF inhibition in the treatment of vasculitis (particularly Wegener's granulomatosis (WG)) are reviewed.

Background

"Tumor necrosis factor" derives its name from properties attributed to the molecule two decades ago: namely, its killing of tumor cells *in vitro*, and its ability to cause hemorrhagic necrosis of malignant growths in mice [11]. Several years later cachectin, a catabolic hormone produced by mouse macrophages, was sequenced and demonstrated to be the same molecule as TNF [12, 13]. The roots of the term "cachectin" (from the Greek *kakos* = "bad" and *hexis* = "condition") illustrate one of the myriad effects of TNF: mediation of the wasting syndromes associated with malignancy, chronic infections, and systemic inflammatory conditions. This TNF effect is achieved through the inhibition of lipoprotein lipase [14].

TNF received notice in the early 1990s for its role as an endogenous mediator of endotoxic shock [15, 16]. The relatively sudden, massive release of TNF characteristic of the sepsis syndrome disrupts the endothelium's inherent anticoagulant properties, activates neutrophils, and induces the release of a host of additional inflammatory cytokines, culminating in cardiovascular collapse. Consequently, the first therapeutic trials of TNF inhibition were directed at sepsis.

Two basic approaches to TNF inhibition were employed in the sepsis syndrome [15–19]: (1) monoclonal antibodies to TNF; and (2) soluble TNF receptor fusion proteins. These two approaches met with similarly disappointing results in sepsis, failing to demonstrate convincing evidence of efficacy despite large studies being conducted. One major sepsis trial actually demonstrated a dose-response relationship between the trial medication and mortality for patients with infections caused by Gram-positive organisms [16].

The failure of TNF inhibition in sepsis probably reflects the tardiness of the intervention with respect to the disease process: because of the fulminant nature of sepsis, irreversible events are often in motion by the time anti-TNF therapy can be administered. In contrast to sepsis, inflammatory conditions such as RA and WG are associated with substantially lower (but *chronically* elevated) levels of TNF. Furthermore, the TNF elevations in these conditions may be confined largely to isolated tissue compartments (e.g., the synovium or kidneys), and levels of TNF may be unmeasurable in the serum.

The consequences of dysfunctional TNF pathways in a wide array of organ systems are now evident. In addition to its role in a variety of autoimmune and inflammatory disorders, TNF contributes to syndromes of insulin resistance [20, 21], wasting [22], bone resorption [23, 24], fever [25], and congestive heart failure [26], among others.

Molecular biology of TNF

The pleiotropic functions of TNF are listed in Table 1. The molecule belongs to a large family of proteins known as TNF ligands. Other members of the TNF ligand family include Fas ligand, CD40 ligand, nerve growth factor, and a host of other proteins known currently (totaling around 20). All members of the TNF ligand family share important structural motifs. For example, most consist of three polypeptide subunits [27]. With the exception of TNF, which exerts its principal effects after secretion by macrophages, most other members of the TNF ligand family are transmembrane proteins, which exert their effects through cell-cell contact. Upon activation, the receptors for these ligands initiate signals for cell proliferation and/or apoptosis (see below), both of which are essential for normal immune system function.

TNF is a homotrimer that is synthesized and expressed as a transmembrane protein. Following expression on the macrophage surface, TNF is cleaved by a converting enzyme known as TACE (TNFα converting enzyme) to produce soluble TNF [28]. Soluble TNF exerts its physiologic and pathologic effects *via* two cell surface

Table 1 - In vivo *functions of tumor necrosis factor*

Bloods vessels	• Alteration of inherent anti-coagulant properties of endothelium
	• Up-regulation of adhesion molecules *via* NF-κB activation
	• Stimulation of angiogenesis
Cells	• Activation of lymphocytes, neutrophils, and platelets
	• Enhancement of CD44's ligand-binding capacity
	• Maturation and migration of dendritic cells into lymphoid organs
	• Proliferation of fibroblasts/synoviocytes
Cytokines, chemokines and other inflammatory mediators:	• Induction of pro-inflammatory
	- cytokines (IL-1, -6, GM-CSF)
	- chemokines (RANTES, IL-8, MIP-1_, MCP-1)
	- prostaglandins, leukotrienes, nitric oxide, reactive oxygen species

receptors, p55 and p75 (these numbers correspond to the molecules' molecular weights, in kDa) [29]. Both receptors are found on virtually every cell type in the body, an indication of the importance of normal TNF pathway function. TNF binds to the extracellular domains of p55 and p75 with equal affinities. Like their TNF ligand, p55 and p75 are part of a larger TNF receptor family that includes approximately 20 presently-known receptors, all of which have similar structures. These receptors are classified into two basic groups based upon the presence or absence of a "death domain" on the cytoplasmic side of the membrane. It is through this death domain that the TNF receptor mediates apoptosis [30].

Of the two TNF receptors, only p55 contains a death domain. The p75 receptor (and other members of the TNF receptor superfamily that do not have death domains) transduces its signal through proteins known as TRAFs, or TNF Receptor Associated Factors [30]. TRAFs induce the production of inflammatory mediators and lead to the proliferation of T lymphocytes *via* activation of the gene transcription factor NF-κB [31].

Each TNF molecule, owing to its trimeric structure, contains three binding sites for the TNFRs. Signal transduction occurs when a molecule of TNF binds and crosslinks two TNF receptors on the surface of the target cell (some of the precise events in this interaction remain to be elucidated). In the absence of ligand attachment and receptor cross-linking, signal transduction does not occur. Soluble TNF receptors result from the proteolytic cleavage of this extracellular domain, an event that is also mediated by TACE. Soluble TNFRs participate in the down-regulation of TNF activity.

Details of the individual functions of the TNFRs p55 and p75 are still incompletely defined, but gene knockout studies in mice [32–34] and variations in the two receptors' cytoplasmic domains – particularly the p55 receptor's death domain [35, 36] – suggest different (but overlapping) functions for these receptors in vivo. Signal transduction by p55 leads principally to apoptosis. In contrast, the consequences of signal transduction by the p75 receptor include cellular proliferation and the production of inflammatory mediators, as well as apoptosis [30]. Triggering of the TNFRs leads to a multitude of pro-inflammatory effects, including the synthesis of IL-1, IL-6, and GM-CSF [31]. TNF also induces the production of matrix metalloproteinases by neutrophils, fibroblasts, and chrondrocytes [37], the elaboration of chemokines (e.g., RANTES, IL-8, MCP-1, and MIP-1α), and the upregulation of adhesion molecule expression [38] (see below).

A closely-related TNF ligand family member that triggers virtually identical biologic responses is known as lymphotoxin-α (LTα, formerly TNFβ). In contrast to the macrophage-derived TNF, LTα is produced exclusively by lymphocytes and natural killer cells. The gene for LTα is tightly linked to the gene for TNF within the major histocompatibility complex, and the two genes share significant homology [39]. LTα binds with comparable affinities to the same two receptors as TNF. As described below, the overlaps in function of these two proteins are potentially relevant to the efficacy (and the side-effects) of specific anti-TNF therapies.

Specific effects of TNF on blood vessels

Among the earliest pathologic changes evident in some forms of vasculitis (e.g., WG) is evidence of an ongoing thrombotic process in the microvasculature [40]. In this regard, the effects of TNF may be directly relevant: the originally-described ability of TNF to induce the necrosis of tumors is secondary to vaso-occlusive changes [11]. Endothelial exposure to TNF tips the delicately-balanced clotting system toward pro-coagulation, stimulating the production of tissue factor and the downregulation of thrombomodulin. Activation of the gene transcription factor NF-κB leads to the expression of several endothelial adhesion molecules, including E-selectin, ICAM-1, and VCAM-1. TNF also alters the sulfation of adhesion receptor CD44 [41], facilitating the migration of circulating lymphocytes through the endothelium and into tissue [31]. In one study [42], treatment of RA with an anti-TNF monoclonal antibody (infliximab; see below) resulted in a dose-dependent decrease in ICAM-1 and E-selectin within hours of medication administration. The reduction of adhesion molecules by this anti-TNF therapy led to decreased synovial infiltration of T lymphocytes [43]. These data indicate that a major disease mechanism of TNF in RA (and probably other diseases) is its activation of vascular endothelium.

Current strategies for the inhibition of TNF

The monoclonal antibody approach: Infliximab

Infliximab (formerly cA2; now Remicade; Centocor; Malvern, PA.) is a chimeric monoclonal antibody comprised of parts of a murine anti-TNF antibody (the variable regions) grafted onto a human $IgG_1\kappa$ molecule (Fig. 1). Thus, the TNF-binding portions of infliximab are murine in origin. The resulting protein, which is approximately two-thirds human, inhibits both cell-associated and secreted TNF [44]. In addition to inhibiting TNF itself, infliximab achieves a multiplicative anti-inflammatory effect by indirectly blocking the production of TNF-dependent cytokines and adhesion molecules [7]. Infliximab may also be cytotoxic to cells within the RA synovium that carry TNF on their cell surfaces, but evidence of massive cell lysis occurring after infliximab administration is absent [7].

Use of infliximab in RA

Most of the anti-TNF trials in RA conducted to date have enrolled patients with severe, refractory disease. In a randomized, double-masked comparison of two dosing regimens of infliximab and placebo, 19 of 24 RA patients (79%) treated with high-dose infliximab (10 mg/kg) responded to treatment within 4 weeks of a single infusion, compared with only two of 24 patients (8%) treated with placebo ($p < 0.0001$) [5]. Eleven of 24 patients (44%) treated with low-dose infliximab (1 mg/kg) achieved similar therapeutic responses, demonstrating a clear dose-response curve for this medication. In this trial, the maximum mean improvement in the number of tender or swollen joints was greater than 60% after only one dose of infliximab.

In an open-label follow-up study to the randomized trial, eight patients received up to four additional infliximab treatments [6]. Although all patients demonstrated magnitudes of response similar to those achieved initially, the durations of response appeared to grow shorter with each successive dose. This observation was attributed to the development of HACA (human anti-chimeric antibodies). To address this problem, subsequent studies of infliximab were performed with methotrexate (MTX) as an adjunct treatment, with the intention of blunting the HACA response.

In a 26-week, double-masked, placebo-controlled trial, 101 patients with active RA were randomized to one of seven groups [7]. The patients received infliximab at doses of 1, 3, or 10 mg/kg, with or without MTX (7.5 mg/week), or placebo plus MTX. Infliximab or placebo was infused at weeks 0, 2, 6, 10, and 14. A 70–90% reduction in the number of swollen and tender joints and in the C-reactive protein was observed throughout the trial for patients who received 10 mg/kg infliximab plus MTX. The co-administration of infliximab and MTX were synergistic at the lowest infliximab dose (1 mg/kg). In that group, MTX prolonged the duration of the ACR20 response [45] to a median of 16.5 weeks ($p < 0.001$ *versus* placebo; $p =$

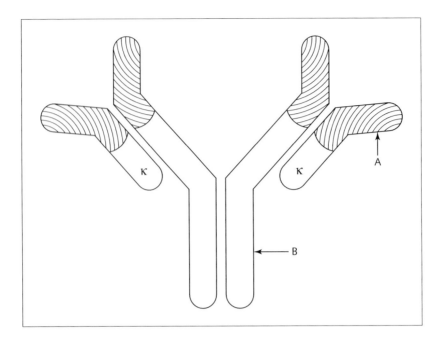

Figure 1
Infliximab is a chimeric monoclonal antibody (approximately two-thirds human) comprised of parts of the variable regions of a murine anti-TNF antibody (A) grafted onto a human IgG$_1$κ molecule (B).

0.006 *versus* no MTX). Concomitant therapy with MTX, even at the low dose of only 7.5 mg/week, also dramatically diminished the appearance of HACA. Data on the immunogenicity of infliximab from this trial suggested that immunologic tolerance to infliximab was induced by higher doses of the medication and potentiated by the simultaneous use of MTX. Among the patients treated with 10 mg/kg of infliximab plus MTX, no HACA responses were reported [7].

Further studies of infliximab, including the recently-completed ATTRACT (Anti-TNF Trial in Rheumatoid Arthritis with Concomitant Therapy) trial [46], have confirmed the promise of infliximab in RA. Infliximab was approved by the United States Food and Drug Administration (FDA) for use in RA in November, 1999. Because of the synergistic effects of infliximab and MTX and the anti-HACA effect of MTX, the use of infliximab in an FDA-approved fashion is contingent on the simultaneous use of MTX.

CDP571 (Celltech Therapeutics, Ltd., UK), a humanized anti-TNF monoclonal antibody consisting of the complementarity determining regions of a murine anti-TNF antibody grafted onto a human IgG$_4$κ molecule, has also been tested in RA

[47]. This genetically-engineered antibody is 95% human. Dose-dependent responses in tender joint counts and pain scores were evident after weeks 1 and 2 in patients receiving the highest CDP571 dose (10 mg/kg). Head-to-head comparisons of infliximab and CDP571 in RA have not been performed.

Use of anti-TNF monoclonal antibodies in Crohn's disease

Crohn's disease, a granulomatous disorder with many pathological similarities to WG, is a chronic inflammatory disorder of the gastrointestinal tract [48]. Infliximab and CDP571 have both demonstrated effectiveness in the management of Crohn's disease, even in patients with treatment-resistant disease. In a trial of infliximab in treatment-resistant Crohn's disease, 65% of the patients responded to a single intravenous dose of infliximab within 1 month, compared with only 17% of patients in the placebo group ($p = 0.001$) [10]. One-third of the patients randomized to infliximab achieved remissions of their disease after only one dose. Infliximab was approved by the FDA for use in Crohn's disease in October, 1998. In a randomized, double-masked, placebo-controlled trial of CDP571, the median Crohn's disease activity score declined by nearly 50% within 2 weeks of a single intravenous CDP571 infusion ($p = 0.0003$) [8]. No significant change in disease activity occurred in the placebo group.

Safety and tolerability of anti-TNF monoclonal antibodies

In approaching the use of anti-TNF monoclonal antibody therapy, there were four issues of paramount concern: (1) the development of anti-HACA; (2) the occurrence of infections; (3) the evolution of autoimmune disorders; and, (4) the possibility of an increase in malignancies. The issue of the HACA response (substantially diminished by concomitant MTX use) was addressed above. The last three concerns will be considered individually below.

Because TNF plays a role in protection against infections [49], increased susceptibility to infections was a major concern about TNF inhibition strategies. In brief, however, more than 5 years of clinical experience with infliximab as a treatment for severe RA and Crohn's disease have demonstrated no such susceptibility, despite careful surveillance. The rate and type of infections that have occurred are similar to those expected in the populations under study.

With regard to autoimmunity, seven of the first 69 RA patients enrolled in infliximab trials (10%) developed anti-dsDNA antibodies [4–6]. Upon follow-up, none of these seven patients developed other clinical features of systemic lupus erythematosus (SLE). In a subsequent multi-dose infliximab study, one patient developed pleuritis and an anti-dsDNA antibody response after the fourth infliximab infusion [7]. Her symptoms responded to moderate doses of corticosteroids, and it is possible that her syndrome represented an SLE-like illness (or drug-induced lupus). The observations of anti-dsDNA antibodies in infliximab-treated patients with RA is intriguing in light of NZB/W mouse studies demonstrating worsening of murine lupus by TNF blockade [50]. Subsequent trials of infliximab have provided reassurance that the induction of classis SLE is not associated with this medication, even though the occurrence of auto-antibodies is fairly common.

Finally, although the question of an increased long-term risk of malignancies cannot be answered with certainty for years to come, the data on this issue to date are encouraging. Among the hundreds of patients enrolled in infliximab trials to date, only a handful of cancers have occurred. The incidence of such malignancies is consistent with the patients' age and other demographic factors. In light of the known pre-disposition of patients with RA to develop particular forms of cancer [51], the failure to observe significant numbers of hematopoietic malignancies is reassuring.

The soluble TNFR fusion protein approach

The other major approach to TNF inhibition is the use of soluble recombinant TNF receptor fusion proteins. To date, these constructs have consisted of molecules created by fusion of the Fc portion of human IgG_1 to two TNFR molecules, either the p75 receptor (etanercept; Enbrel; Immunex Corporation; Seattle, WA.) or the p55 (lenercept; Ro-45-2081; Hoffman-LaRoche; Basel, Switzerland).

Etanercept (Fig. 2) is a dimeric fusion protein produced by linking the human DNA encoding the p75 TNFR to the DNA template for the Fc portion of human IgG_1. This DNA-linked product is then inserted into a mammalian expression vector [52]. The resulting protein (which, unlike infliximab, contains only human amino acid sequences), binds two TNF molecules. The dimeric nature of etanercept affords superior binding affinity (up to 50-fold) and TNF-neutralizing capacity (approximately 1000-fold) compared to the native monomeric TNFR. The Fc moiety, which contains the hinge region as well as the C_H2 and C_H3 domains of IgG_1, extends the molecule's circulating half-life from only a few minutes to approximately 96 h.

Etanercept is postulated to exert its anti-TNF effects *via* several mechanisms [53]:

- Competitive inhibition of binding by TNF to the native TNF receptors that reside on the surfaces of inflammatory cells
- Acting as a cytokine "carrier" for TNF, rendering it biologically unavailable even though it prolongs the molecule's serum half-life
- Modulation of biological events mediated by "downstream" molecules, whose functions are regulated by TNF. For example, in RA, etanercept decreases the levels of IL-1, IL-6, E-selectin, and ICAM-1
- Finally, in addition to binding TNF, etanercept binds and disrupts the function of $LT\alpha$ [30].

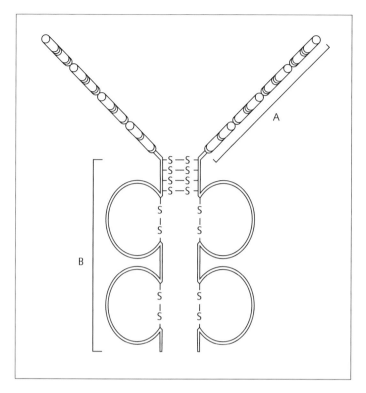

Figure 2
Etanercept is a dimeric fusion protein produced by linking the human DNA encoding the p75 TNFR (A) to the DNA template for the Fc portion of human IgG$_1$ (B). The resulting protein binds two TNF molecules.

A 3-month trial of etanercept in 180 patients with refractory RA confirmed the efficacy of this medication [1]. Seventy-five percent of patients receiving the highest dose of etanercept (16 mg/m^2) achieved at least a 20% ACR clinical response, compared with 14% in the placebo group ($p < 0.001$). The mean percent reduction in the number of tender or swollen joints was 61% in the 16 mg/m^2, compared with 25% in the placebo group ($p = 0.001$). The time to response among patients treated with etanercept was swift: generally 4 weeks in the 16 mg/m^2 group. A dose-response curve was evident as etanercept doses increased from 0.25 mg/m^2 b.i.w. to 2 mg/m^2 b.i.w. to 16 mg/m^2 b.i.w. Following the cessation of therapy at 3 months, patients' inflammatory arthritis promptly returned.

These findings were extended in a Phase III trial involving 234 RA patients who had failed a series of disease-modifying agents [2]. In that trial, the patients were randomized to receive either placebo or 10 or 25 mg of etanercept b.i.w. (the last dose corresponding to 16 mg/m^2). Ninety percent of the patients enrolled had failed MTX treatment before entering the trial, illustrating the severity of their disease. Nevertheless, at 6 months, 59% of the patients in the 25 mg etancercept group and 51% in the 10 mg etanercept group had responded, contrasted with only 11% of the patients in the placebo group ($p < 0.001$). In the 25 mg etancercept group, the mean percentage reduction in the number of tender and swollen joints at 6 months was 56% and 47%, respectively, compared with 6% and –7% in the placebo group ($p < 0.05$). In open-label extension trials, durable responses to etanercept have been shown for up to two years.

In an additional Phase III trial investigating patients with refractory RA, etanercept was proven to be safe when used in conjunction with MTX [3]. Seventy-one percent of the patients treated with etanercept/MTX responded to therapy (compared with 27% in the placebo/MTX group, $p < 0.001$). Using the more rigorous ACR50 standard, the response rates were 39% and 3% in the etanercept and placebo groups, respectively ($p < 0.001$).

Responses to etanercept were not confined to clinical measures of arthritis severity. Rather, patients also reported dramatic improvements in quality of life, as measured by the Health Assessment Questionnaire (HAQ) [54]. The Disability, Vitality, Mental Health, and General Health Status subdomains of the HAQ improved among etanercept-treated patients compared to controls. The perception of General Health Status among etanercept-treated patients, for example, improved by 50% over 12 months. Over the same time period, the General Health Status perception of placebo-treated patients declined by 2% [3].

Use of etanercept in other rheumatic conditions

The success of etanercept in the treatment of RA has been extended to other forms of inflammatory arthritis. The medication is efficacious in juvenile RA [55], and was approved by the FDA for that indication in 1999. A recently-completed randomized trial of 60 patients with psoriatic arthritis demonstrated results that are strikingly similar to those in RA with regard to the achievement of ACR20, ACR50, and ACR70 responses [56].

Safety and tolerability of etanercept

Because etanercept contains only human amino acid sequences, concerns about immunogenicity of the medication are substantially fewer compared to the chimeric monoclonal antibody infliximab. Indeed, throughout Phase I, II, and III studies with the medication, clinically significant antibody formation against etanercept did not occur [1, 3]. Among the first 578 patients with RA tested in clinical trials of etanercept, antibodies to the medication were found in only six. None of the antibodies in those six patients had drug-neutralizing activity.

The inhibition of LTα as well as TNF by etanercept has raised theoretical concerns regarding the possibility of increased side-effects compared to infliximab. However, with regard to specific potential adverse events (e.g., the risks of infection and malignancies), etanercept has demonstrated a safety record comparable to that of infliximab. No substantive problems have emerged to date. Post-marketing surveillance data detected the occurrence of 25 serious infections and six deaths due to infection in patients using etanercept, but close inspection revealed that most of these patients had multiple co-morbidities pre-disposing them to infections, and some had active infections of leg ulcers at the time etanercept was begun. The current FDA recommendation is that the use of etanercept be postponed or suspended in the presence of an active infection.

A fusion protein failure: the case of lenercept

During the mid-1990s lenercept, a glycosylated fusion protein consisting of two human p55 TNFRs linked to the Fc portion of human IgG$_1$, was investigated for use in RA [57–59]. In contrast to the dramatic effectiveness of etanercept in RA, clinical trials of lenercept were halted because of the frequent occurrence of side-effects and reports of disease worsening [58, 59]. In one open-label extension trial, 30 of the 63 patients enrolled (48%) dropped out of the study (21 for lack of efficacy). The full implications of these strikingly different results with these different soluble fusion proteins remain unclear.

Use of anti-TNF strategies in vasculitis

The remarkable effectiveness of some anti-TNF strategies in inflammatory arthritis and Crohn's disease enhances their appeal as a treatment for vasculitis. Compelling evidence suggests that anti-TNF strategies may be effective in the vasculitides, particularly in granulomatous forms of these diseases.

Rationale for use in the vasculitides

The following pieces of evidence suggest that TNF plays a major role in WG, and that an anti-TNF strategy may be effective in this disease:

- Granuloma formation – the pathologic hallmark of the disease – is inhibited completely by the absence of TNF [60].
- Active WG is associated with a dramatically upregulated Th1 cytokine pathway, a pathway in which the role of TNF is pivotal [61].
- Transcription of the TNF gene is enhanced in peripheral blood mononuclear cells from patients with WG [62]. CD4$^+$ T cells from patients with WG produce ele-

vated levels of TNF [61].

- Serum levels of both TNF and its soluble receptors, p55 and p75, are elevated in patients with active WG [63, 64]. Levels of p55, an excellent surrogate for TNF levels, correlate with WG activity as measured by the Birmingham Vasculitis Activity Score [63]. With the induction of remission, levels of these molecules normalize.
- Immunohistochemistry, polymerase chain reaction, and *in situ* hybridization studies of renal biopsies from patients with WG confirm that TNF-positive cells (now known to be macrophages) infiltrate histologically active renal lesions. Such cells are also present within the walls of arteries and arterioles in acute vasculitic lesions [65].
- Neutrophils are important in the pathophysiology of WG. *In vitro* priming of activated neutrophils with TNF markedly enhances the ability of ANCA to stimulate neutrophil degranulation, fueling the leukocytoclastic vasculitis associated with this disorder [66-68].
- In most studies, a distinctive feature of WG is its strong association with the ANCA response to proteinase 3 (PR3), a constituent of neutrophil granules. TNF synergistically induces PR3 expression on both neutrophils (and possibly endothelial cells). TNF also facilitates the presentation of PR3 by macrophages [69–71]. These actions increase the accessibility of PR3 for binding with ANCA, and may therefore contribute directly to the pathophysiology of WG in most patients.

A phase I trial in Wegener's granulomatosis

Interim results of a 6-month, open-label trial of etanercept in WG are now available [72]. Between March and July 1999, 20 patients with active WG were enrolled in this preliminary study, designed to evaluate the safety of etanercept in WG. In addition to standard medications for WG, etanercept was administered subcutaneously at a dose of 25 mg twice a week. Though not the principal aim of the trial, the efficacy of this approach was assessed by a WG-specific modification of the Birmingham Vasculitis Activity Score (BVAS [73]) known as BVAS for WG [74].

Evidence of active WG included a diverse array of anatomic sites and clinical manifestations at trial entry (Tab. 2). Standard medications employed at the time of entry (administered according to severity of disease) included prednisone in 17 patients (85%), cyclophosphamide in six (30%), MTX in 9 (45%), azathioprine in three (15%), and cyclosporine in one (5%). Etanercept was added as the only new treatment variable in 14 (70%) of the patients enrolled.

An interim analysis was conducted at a mean of 21 weeks of treatment (range: 9–28 weeks). At the time of this analysis, all 20 patients (100%) remained on etanercept. Without exception, the medication was well-tolerated. Injection site reactions, so common in trials of RA patients, were uncommon at the time of interim

*Table 2 - Patient characteristics at entry: open-label trial of etanercept in Wegener's granu-
lomatosis (WG) (n = 20).*

Male : female ratio	9 : 11
Mean age (years)	46.7 (25–73)
Mean Birmingham vasculitis activity score for WG	3.7 (range 1–8)
Sites of disease:	
Upper respiratory tract	16 (80%)
Arthritis	9 (45%)
Conductive hearing loss	4 (20%)
Glomerulonephritis	4 (20%)
Pulmonary nodules/endobronchial disease	3 (15%)
Orbital mass	2 (10%)
Mesenteric vasculitis	2 (10%)
Meningeal involvement	2 (10%)
Cutaneous vasculitis	2 (10%)
Alveolar hemorrhage	1 (5%)
Fever	1 (5%)
Overwhelming fatigue	1 (5%)
Conjunctivitis	1 (5%)

analysis (one patient had one injection site reaction). In addition, despite the substantial use of concomitant immunosuppression, there were few infections. Only one major infection occurred – a case of pneumococcal pneumonia in a patient with severe subglottic stenosis and concomitant treatment with cyclophosphamide and corticosteroids. This patient's infection was uncomplicated, responding promptly to antibiotics. Etanercept was continued. Other adverse events, including all-cause hospitalizations, cytopenias, and hepato-renal dysfunction, have not occurred with unusual frequencies, and have not been attributed to etanercept.

In terms of efficacy, the results at the interim analysis were as follows. The mean BVAS for WG at entry was 3.7 (range 1–8) (one point scored for a "minor" disease manifestation, three for a "major") [74]. Upon follow-up at a mean of 21 weeks of treatment, the mean BVAS for WG score was 0.9 (range 0–4) ($p < 0.001$; 95% confidence interval: 2.1–3.5). Comparing the first to the last BVAS for WG assessment, 19 (95%) of the patients had improved, including 14 of 14 in whom etanercept was added as the only new treatment variable. 16 of the 20 patients (80%) achieved BVAS for WG scores of zero at some point during follow-up. Improvement in constitutional symptoms was nearly universal among patients in this trial.

Although responses to the treatment regimen (which included both etanercept and standard of care medications) were the rule, limited disease flares and persistent minor features of active disease were also common. Seven minor disease flares, principally upper respiratory tract manifestations, had occurred at the time of the interim analysis. One major disease flare occurred (a case of glomerulonephritis).

In this unrandomized trial in which standard medications were used simultaneously with etanercept, it is not possible to objectively assess the effectiveness of etanercept in WG. However, results of the trial to date appear to confirm the safety of etanercept in WG (even when the TNF inhibitor is combined with immunosuppressive medications), and provide sound rationale for the conduct of a randomized, placebo-controlled trial of etanercept in this disease.

Issues in the design of a randomized, multi-center trial in WG

Experience with the treatment of WG over the past 30 years using the combination of corticosteroids and "cytotoxic" agents (e.g., cyclophosphamide or methotrexate) has repeatedly demonstrated several points [72, 75–77]. First, corticosteroids alone are insufficient to treat WG in most cases, and combined approaches consisting of corticosteroids plus a cytotoxic agent are required. Second, if used in a timely and judicious fashion, such conventional therapy is effective in inducing remission in a high percentage of cases (approximately 80% or higher). Third, this conventional approach to treatment, though effective, is associated with substantial toxicities that ultimately limit the doses that can be used safely. Fourth, WG has a propensity to flare as conventional therapies are tapered. In a large series of patients followed at the NIH, for example, only 38% of patients treated with corticosteroids and oral daily cyclophosphamide achieved durable remissions with their initial courses of treatment [75]. Thus, the most vexing issue today confronting patients with this form of vasculitis is the absence of a well-tolerated, effective medication for the maintenance of disease remission.

A randomized, double-blind, placebo-controlled trial of etanercept in WG is now under way in the United States. The principal aim of the Wegener's Granulomatosis Etanercept Trial (WGET) is to test the efficacy of etanercept in the maintenance of disease remissions. In addition to either etanercept or placebo, all patients will receive standard medications for their disease at the time of trial entry. Those with limited WG will receive methotrexate and corticosteroids, and those with severe WG will receive cyclophosphamide and corticosteroids. After the patients' disease is controlled with therapy (i.e., the standard medications plus either etanercept or placebo), the standard medications will be tapered according to regimens designed to insure patient safety, diminish morbidity associated with the standard medications, and test the efficacy of etanercept in sustaining disease remissions. The treat-

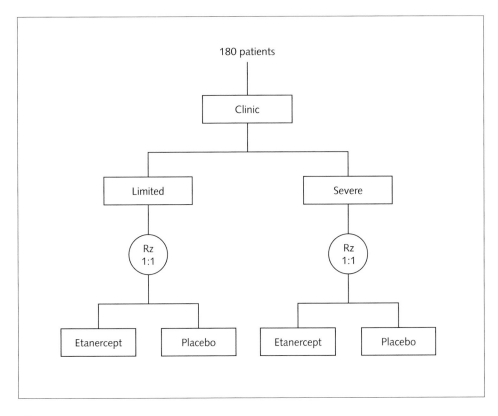

Figure 3
Randomization scheme for the Wegener's Granulomatosis Etanercept Trial. Following strat-
ification by clinic (center) and disease severity (limited versus severe), patients are random-
ized to receive either etanercept or placebo in a 1:1 ratio. All patients in the trial receive
standard therapies for WG: those with limited disease receive methotrexate and cortico-
steroids; those wih severe disease receive cyclophosphamide and corticosteroids. Standard
therapies are tapered according to protocol after the achievement of remission.

ment allocation scheme for this trial is depicted in Figure 3, and additional features
of this trial are outlined below:

Type of study
- Randomized, parallel treatment design.
- Placebo-controlled.
- Multi-center (eight clinical centers in the United States).

Enrollment
- 30 months enrollment period. Total enrollment goal (see sample size, below) will require an enrollment rate of nine patients per clinic per year.

Length of treatment
- Last patient enrolled to be followed for a minimum of 12 months on treatment.
- Common closing date of trial on this date (i.e., all patients have the same completion date).

Masking
- Patients and clinic personnel unaware of treatment assignments.
- Data and Safety Monitoring Board and biostatisticians not masked.

Stratification
- By clinic.
- By disease severity (limited versus severe).

Treatment groups
- Etanercept (25 mg/dose), injected subcutaneously twice a week.
- Placebo, injected subcutaneously twice a week.
- 1:1 allocation ratio.

Other medications
- Corticosteroids plus either methotrexate or cyclophosphamide.
- Standard medications tapered according to protocol based on published guidelines.

Outcomes
- Primary: Rate of achievement and maintenance of remission in the two treatment groups. Remission assessed by BVAS for WG.
- Pre-specified secondary outcomes related to disease- and treatment-specific events.

Data collection schedule
- Year 1: Trial entry; 6 weeks; then at 3, 6, 9, and 12 months.
- Subsequently: every 3 months until the common closeout.

Sample size
- Total sample size: 180 patients (90 patients in each arm).
- Parameter assumptions:
  - Principal outcome measure is the percentage of patients who achieve sustained missions during followup. A sustained remission is defined as remission for at least 6 months, i.e., three consecutive visits with a BVAS score of 0.
  - Two-sided chi-square tests.
  - $\alpha = 0.05$ (two-sided).
  - $\beta = 0.20$ (power = 80%).
  - Allowance for 15% decrease in sample size due to patient dropout, loss to follow-up, and heterogeneity of effect associated with disease severity.
- Minimum detectable difference between groups ranges from 15% to 22%.

Data analysis and monitoring
- Primary analyses by original treatment assignment (intention-to-treat).
- Include all randomized patients and all events occurring after randomization.
- Secondary analyses consisting of all patients who complete trial.
- Interim analyses for safety and efficacy planned.

The future of anti-cytokine strategies for vasculitis

Anti-TNF strategies may also have extensions to other forms of vasculitis, particularly those associated with granulomatous inflammation or ANCAs. The possible role of TNF in a wide variety of non-granulomatous, non-ANCA associated vasculitides requires further study. The inflammatory process associated with vasculitis involves a complex array of cytokines, and optimal treatment may include combinations of anti-cytokine strategies. Testing of these approaches in a rigorous fashion will be challenging, and will probably require international collaboration.

In addition to the currently available TNF inhibitors described in this chapter, additional TNF inhibitors are in earlier stages of clinical development. These approaches include inhibitors of TACE (the enzyme that cleaves TNF from the cell surface of macrophages), inhibitors of phosphodiesterase IV (which regulates TNF production), and gene transfer strategies, predicated upon manipulations leading to overexpression of TNF receptors [78–80].

The first decade of this millennium holds promise for significant advances in the treatment of the vasculitis. Developments in molecular biology will equip researchers with an expanding array of tools to investigate the etiology and immunopathogenesis of inflammatory disorders. In addition, growing interest in the vasculitides in recent years has fostered multi-center collaborations on an unprecedented scale, both in Europe and in the United States.

References

1   Moreland LW, Baumgartner SW, Schiff MH, Tindall EA, Fleischmann RM, Weaver AL, Ettlinger RE, Cohen S, Koopman WJ, Mohler K et al (1997) Treatment of rheumatoid arthritis with a recombinant human tumor necrosis factor receptor (p75)-Fc fusion protein. *N Engl J Med* 337: 141–147

2   Moreland LW, Schiff MH, Baumgartner SW, Tindall EA, Fleischmann RM, Bulpitt KJ, Weaver AL, Keystone EC, Furst DE, Mease PJ et al (1999) Etanercept therapy in rheumatoid arthritis: A randomized, controlled trial. *Ann Intern Med* 130: 478–486

3   Weinblatt ME, Kremer JM, Bankhurst AD, Bulpitt KJ, Fleischmann RM, Fox RI, Jackson CG, Lange M, Burge DJ (1999) A trial of Etanercept, a recombinant tumor necrosis factor receptor:Fc fusion protein, in patients with rheumatoid arthritis receiving methotrexate. *N Engl J Med* 340: 253–259

4   Elliott MJ, Maini RN, Feldman M, Long-Fox A, Charles P, Katsikis P, Brennan FM, Walker J, Bijl H, Ghrayeb J et al (1993) Treatment of rheumatoid arthritis with chimeric monoclonal antibodies to tumor necrosis factor α. *Arthritis Rheum* 36: 1681–1690

5   Elliott MJ, Maini RN, Feldmann M, Kalden JR, Antoni C, Smolen JS (1994) Randomised double-blind comparison of chimeric monoclonal antibody to tomour necrosis factor α (cA2) versus placebo in rheumatoid arthritis. *Lancet* 344: 1105–1110

6   Elliott MJ, Maini RN, Feldmann M, Long-Fox A, Charles P, Bijl H, Woody JN (1994) Repeated therapy with monoclonal antibody to tumor necrosis factor a (cA2) in patients with rheumatoid arthritis. *Lancet* 344: 1125–1127

7   Maini RN, Breedveld FC, Kalden JR, Smolen JS, Davis D, MacFarlane JD, Antoni C, Leeb B, Elliott MJ, Woody JN et al (1998) Therapeutic efficacy of multiple intravenous infusions of anti-tumor necrosis factor α monoclonal antibody combined with low-dose weekly methotrexate in rheumatoid arthritis. *Arthritis Rheum* 41: 1552–1563

8   Stack W, Mann S, Roy A, Heath P, Sopwith M, Freeman J et al (1997) Randomised controlled trial of CDP571 antibody to tumour necrosis factor-α in Crohn's disease. *Lancet* 349: 521–524

9   Targan S, Landers C, Vidrich A, Czaja A (1995) High-titer antineutrophil cytoplasmic antibodies in type-1 autoimmune hepatitis. *Gastroenterol* 108: 1159–1166

10 Targan S, Hanauer S, van Deventer S, Mayer L, Present DH, Braakman T, De Woody KL, Schaible TF, Rutgeerts PJ (1997) A short-term study of chimeric monoclonal antibody cA2 to tumor necrosis factor a for Crohn's disease. *N Engl J Med* 337: 1029–1035

11 Carswell E, Old L, Kassel R, Green S, Fiore N, Williamson B (1975) An endotoxin-induced serum factor that causes necrosis of tumors. *Proc Natl Acad Sci USA* 75: 3666–3670

12 Beutler B, Mahoney J, Le Trang N, Pekala P, Cerami A (1985) Purification of cachectin, a lipoprotein lipase-supressing hormone secreted by endotoxin-induced RAW 264.7 cells. *J Exp Med* 161: 984–995

13 Beutler B, Greenwald D, Hulmes J, Chang M, Pan YC, Mathison J, Ulevitch R, Cerami

A (1985) Identity of tumour necrosis factor and the macrophage-secreted factor cachectin. *Nature* 316: 552–554

14 Kawakami M, Pekala P, Lane M, Cerami A (1982) Lipoprotein lipase suppression in 3T3-L1 cells by an endotoxin-induced mediator from exudates cells. *Proc Natl Acad Sci USA* 79: 912–916

15 Wherry J, Pennington J, Wenzel R (1993) Tumor necrosis factor and the therapeutic potential of anti-tumor necrosis factor antibodies. *Crit Care Med* 21: S436–S440

16 Fisher CJ, Agosti JM, Opal SM, Lowry SF, Balk RA, Sadoff JC, Abraham E, Schein RMH, Benjamin E (1996) Treatment of septic shock with the tumor necrosis factor receptor:Fc fusion protein. The Soluble TNF Receptor Sepsis Study Group. *N Engl J Med* 334: 1697–1702

17 van der Poll T, Lowry S (1995) Tumour necrosis factor in sepsis: Mediator of multiple organ failure or essential part of host defense? *Shock* 3: 1–12

18 Agosti J, Fisher C, Opal S, Lowry S, Balk R, Sadoff J (1994) Treatment of patients with sepsis syndrome with soluble TNF receptor (sTNFR). *Proc 34th Annual ICAAC* 34: 65

19 Abraham E, Wunderink R, Silverman H, Perl TM, Nasraway S, Levy H, Bone R, Wenzel RP, Balk R, Allred R et al (1995) Efficacy and safety of monoclonal antibody to human tumor necrosis factor alpha in patients with sepsis syndrome: a randomized, double-blind, multicenter clinical trial. *JAMA* 273: 934–941

20 Hotamisligil G, Arner P, Caro J, Atkinson R, Spiegelman B (1995) Increased adipose tissue expression of tumor necrosis factor alpha in human obesity and insulin resistance. *J Clin Invest* 95: 2409–2415

21 Hotamisligil G (1999) The role of TNF-alpha and TNF receptors in obesity and insulin resistance. *J Intern Med* 245: 621–625

22 Spiegelman B, Hotamisligil G (1993) Through thick and thin: wasting, obesity, and TNF alpha. *Cell* 73: 625–627

23 Bertolini D, Nedwin G, Bringman T, Smith D, Mundy G (1986) Stimulation of bone resorption and inhibition of bone formation *in vitro* by human necrosis factor. *Nature* 319: 516–518

24 Saklatvala J (1986) Tumour necrosis factor a stimulates resorption and inhibits synthesis of proteoglycan in cartilage. *Nature* 322: 547–549

25 Dinarello C (1999) Cytokines as endogenous pyrogens. *J Infect Dis* 179 (Suppl 2): S294–304

26 Torre-Amione G, Bozkurt B, Deswal A, Mann D (1999) An overview of tumor necrosis factor alpha and the failing heart. *Curr Opin Cardiol* 14: 206–210

27 Bazzoni F, Beutler B (1996) The tumor necrosis factor ligand and receptor families. *N Engl J Med* 334: 1717–1725

28 Tracey K, Vlassara H, Cerami A (1989) Cachectin/tumor necrosis factor. *Lancet* 1: 1126

29 Banner DW, D'Arcy A, Janes W, Gentz R, Schoenfeld HJ, Broger C, Loetscher H, Lesslauer W (1993) Crystal structure of the soluble human 55 kd TNF receptor-human TNF beta complex: implications for TNF receptor activation. *Cell* 73: 341–345

30 Beutler B, Bazzoni F (1998) TNF, apoptosis and autoimmunity: A common thread? *Blood, Cells, Molecules and Disease* 24: 216–230

31 Fujisawa K, Aono H, Hasunuma T, Yamamoto K, Mita S, Nishioka K (1996) Activation of transcription factor NF-KB in human synovial cells in response to tumor necrosis factor α. *Arthritis Rheum* 39: 197–203

32 Pfeffer K, Matsuyama T, Kündig TM, Wakeham A, Kishihara K, Shahinian A, Wiegmann K, Ohashi PS, Kronke M, Mak TW (1993) Mice deficient for the 55kD tumor necrosis factor receptor are resistant to endotoxic shock, yet succumb to *L. monocytogenes* infection. *Cell* 73: 457–467

33 Rothe M, Wong S, Henzel W, Goeddel D (1994) A novel family of putative signal transducers associated with the cytoplasmic domain of the 75 kD tumor necrosis factor receptor. *Cell* 78: 681–692

34 Erickson SL, de Sauvage FJ, Kikly K, Carver-Moore K, Pitts-Meek S, Gillett N, Sheehan KC, Schreiber RP, Goeddel DV, Moore MW (1994) Decreased sensitivity to tumour necrosis factor but normal T-cell development in TNF receptor-2-deficient mice. *Nature* 372: 560–563

35 Tartaglia L, Ayres T, Wong G, Goeddel D (1993) A novel domain within the 55 kd TNF receptor signals cell death. *Cell* 74: 845–853

36 Ashkenazi A, Dixit V (1998) Death receptors: signaling and modulation. *Science* 281: 1305–1308

37 Jones R, Moreland L (1999) Tumor necrosis factor inhibitors for rheumatoid arthritis. *Bulletin Rheum Diseases* 48: 1–4

38 Carlos T, Harlan J (1994) Leukocyte-endothelial adhesion molecules. *Blood* 84: 2068–2101

39 Pennica D, Nedwin J, Hayflick P, Seeburg PH, Derynck R, Palladino MA, Kohr WJ, Aggarwal BB, Goeddel DV (1984) Human tumor necrosis factor: precursor structure, expression, and homology to lymphotoxin. *Nature* 312: 724–729

40 Wegener F (1990) Wegener's granulomatosis: Thoughts and observations of a pathologist. *Eur Arch Otorhinolaryngol* 247: 133–142

41 Maiti A, Maki G, Johnson P (1998) TNF-alpha induction of CD44-mediated leukocyte adhesion by sulfation. *Science* 282: 941–943

42 Paleolog E, Hunt M, Elliott M, Feldmann M, Maini R, Woody J (1996) Deactivation of vascular endothelium by monoclonal anti-tumor necrosis factor α antibody in rheumatoid arthritis. *Arthritis Rheum* 39: 1082–1091

43 Tak PP, Taylor PC, Breedveld FC, Smeets TJM, Daha M, Kluin PM, Meinders AE, Maini RN (1996) Decrease in cellularity and expression of adhesion molecules by anti-tumor necrosis factor α monoclonal antibody in patients with rheumatoid arthritis. *Arthritis Rheum* 39: 1077–1081

44 Feldmann M, Elliott M, Woody J, Maini RN (1997) Anti-tumor necrosis factor-α therapy of rheumatoid arthritis. *Adv Immunol* 64: 283–350

45 Felson DT, Anderson JJ, Boers M, Bombardier C, Furst D, Goldsmith C, Katz LM,

Lightfoot R Jr, Paulus H, Strand V (1995) American College of Rheumatology. Preliminary definition of improvement in rheumatoid arthritis. *Arthritis Rheum* 38: 727–735

46 Lipsky P, St. Clair W, Kavanaugh A, McCune W, Smolen J, Breedveld F, Furst D, Kalden J, Weissman M, Braakman T et al (1998) Long-term control of signs and symptoms of rheumatoid arthritis with chimeric monoclonal anti-TNF-α antibody (infliximab) in patients with active disease on methotrexate. *Arthritis Rheum* 41: S364

47 Rankin ECC, Choy EHS, Kassimos D, Kingsley GH, Sopwith AM, Isenberg DA, Panayi (1995) The therapeutic effects of an engineered human anti-tumour necrosis factor alpha antibody (CDP571) in rheumatoid arthritis. *Br J Rheum* 34: 334–342

48 Podolsky D (1991) Inflammatory bowel disease. *N Engl J Med* 325: 928–938

49 Vassalli P (1992) The pathophysiology of tumor necrosis factors. *Ann Rev Immunol* 10: 411–452

50 Jacob C, McDevitt H (1988) Tumour necrosis factor-alpha in murine autoimmune "lupus" nephritis. *Nature* 331: 356–358

51 Bannworth B, Vernhes J, Schaeverbeke T, Dehais J (1995) The facts about methotrexte in rheumatoid arthritis. *Rev Rheum* 62: 471–473

52 Peppel K, Crawford D, Beutler B (1991) A tumor necrosis factor receptor- IgG heavy chain chimeric protein as a bivalent antagonist of TNF activity. *J Exp Med* 174: 1483–1489

53 Mohler KM, Torrance DS, Smith CA, Goodwin RG, Stremler KE, Fung VP, Madani H, Widmer MB (1993) Soluble tumor necrosis factor receptors are effective therapeutic agents in lethal endotoxemia and function simultaneously as both TNF carriers and TNF antagonists. *J Immunol* 151: 1548

54 Ramey D, Fries J, Singh G (1996) The Health Assesment Questionnaire 1995 – status and review. In: B Spilker (ed): *Quality of life and pharmacoeconomics in clinical trials*. Lippincott-Raven, Philadelphia

55 Lovell DJ, Giannini EH, Reiff A, Cawkwell GD, Silverman ED, Nocton JJ, Stein LD, Gedalia A, Ilowite NT, Wallace CA et al (2000) Etanercept in children with polyarticular juvenile rheumatoid arthritis. *N Engl J Med* 342 (11): 763–769

56 Mease P, Goffe B, Metz J, Vanderstoep A (1999) Enbrel (Etanercept) in patients with psoriatic arthritis and psoriasis. *Arthritis Rheum* 42: S377

57 Sander O, Rau R, vanRiel P, vandePutte L, Hasler F, Baudin M, Lüdin E, McAuliffe T, Dickinson S, Kähny M-R et al (1996) Neutralization of TNF by lenercept (TNFR55-IgG1, Ro 45-2081) in patients with rheumatoid arthritis treated for 3 months: results of a European phase II trial. *Arthritis Rheum* 39 (9 Suppl): S1288

58 Hasler F, van de Putte L, Dumont E, Kneer J, Bock J, Dickinson S, Lesslauer W, Van der Auwera P (1996) Safety and efficacy of the neutralization by lenercept (TNFR55-IgG1, Ro 45-2081) in patients with rheumatoid arthritis exposed to a single dose. *Arthritis Rheum* 39 (9 Suppl): S1291

59 Hasler F, van de Putte L, Baudin M, Lüdin E, Durrwell L, McAuliffe T, Van der Auwera P (1996) Chronic TNF neutralization (up to 1 year) by lenercept (TNFR55-IgG1, Ro

45-2081) in patients with rheumatoid arthritis: Results of an open-label extension of a double-blind single dose phase I study. *Arthritis Rheum* 39 (9 Suppl): S1292

60   Kindler V, Sappino A, Grau G, Piguet P, Vassalli P (1989) The inducing role of tumor necrosis factor in the development of bactericidal granulomas during BCG infection. *Cell* 56: 731–740

61   Ludviksson BR, Sneller MC, Chua KS, Talar-Williams C, Langford CA, Ehrhardt RO, Fauci AS, Strober W (1998) Active Wegener's granulomatosis is associated with HLA-DR⁺ CD4⁺ T cells exhibiting an unbalanced Th1-Type T cell cytokine pattern: Reversal with IL-10. *J Immun* 160: 3602–3609

62   Deguchi Y, Shibata N, Kishimoto S (1990) Enhanced expression of the tumour necrosis factor/cachectin gene in peripheral blood mononuclear cells from patients with systemic vasculitis. *Clin Exp Immunol* 81: 311–314

63   Nassonov EL, Samsonov MY, Tilz GP, Beketova ZV, Semenkova EN, Baranov A, Wachter H, Fuchs D (1997) Serum concentrations of neopterin, soluble interleukin 2 receptor, and doluble tumor necrosis factor receptor in Wegener's granulomatosis. *J Rheum* 24: 666–670

64   Jonasdottir O, Bendtzen K, Skjodt H, Petersen J (1998) Elevated serum levels of soluble tumor necrosis factor receptors in Wegener's granulomatosis. *Arthritis Rheum* 41: S503

65   Noronha I, Kruger C, Andrassy K, Ritz E, Waldherr R (1993) *In situ* production of TNF-alpha, IL-1 beta and IL-2R in ANCA-positive glomerulonephritis. *Kidney International* 43: 682–692

66   Falk R, Hogan S, Carey T, Jennette J, Network G (1990) Clinical course of anti-neutrophil cytoplasmic autoantibody-associated glomerulonephritis and systemic vasculitis. *Ann Intern Med* 11: 656–663

67   Falk R, Terrell R, Charles L, Jennette J (1990) Anti-neutrophil cytoplasmic autoantibodies induce neutrophils to degranulate and produce oxygen radicals *in vitro*. *Proc Natl Acad Sci USA* 87: 4115–4119

68   Reumaux D, Vossebeld P, Roos D, Verhoeven A (1995) Effect of tumor necrosis factor-induced integrin activation on Fc gamma receptor II-mediated signal transduction: relevance for activation of neutrophils by anti-proteinase 3 or anti-myeloperoxidase antibodies. *Blood* 86: 3189–3195

69   Mayet W, Meyer Zum Buschenfelde K (1993) Antibodies to proteinase 3 increase adhesion of neutrophils to human endothelial cells. *Clin Exp Immunol* 94: 440–446

70   Csernok E, Ernst M, Scmitt W, Bainton D, Gross W (1994) Activated neutrophils express proteinase 3 on their plasma membrane *in vitro* and *in vivo*. *Clin Exp Immunol* 98: 244–250

71   Ralston D, Marsh C, Lowe M, Wewers M (1997) Antineutrophil cytoplasmic antibodies induce monocyte IL-8 release. *J Clin Invest* 100: 1416–1424

72   Stone JH, Hellmann DB, Uhlfelder ML, Bedocs NM, Crook SL, Hoffman GS (2001) Etanercept in Wegener's granulomatosis (WG): Results of an open-label trial. *Arthritis Rheum* 44 (5): 1149–1154

73   Luqmani RA, Bacon PA, Moots RJ, Janssen BA, Pall A, Emery P, Savage C, Adu D

(1994) Birmingham Vasculitis Activity Score (BVAS) in systemic necrotizing vasculitis. *Q J Med* 87: 671–678

74   INSSYS (The International Network for the Study of Systemic Vasculitides) (1999) Vasculitis Activity Score for Wegener's granulomatosis: A report from the International Network for Study of the Systemic Vasculitides. *Arthritis Rheum* 42: S317

75   Hoffman GS, Kerr GS, Leavitt RY, Hallahan CW, Lebovics RS, Travis WD, Rottem M, Fauci AS (1992) Wegener's granulomatosis: An analysis of 158 patients. *Ann Intern Med* 116: 488–498

76   Guillevin L, Cordier J-F, Lhote F, Cohen, Pascal, Jarrousse B, Royer I, Lesavre P, Jacquot C, Bindi P, Bielefeld P et al (1997) A prospective, multicenter, randomized trial comparing steroids and pulse cyclophosphamide versus steroids and oral cyclophosphamide in the treatment of generalized Wegener's granulomatosis. *Arthritis Rheum* 40: 2187–2198

77   Sneller MC, Hoffmann GS, Talar-Williams C, Kerr GS, Hallahan CW, Fauci AS (1995) An analysis of forty-two Wegener's granulomatosis patients treated with methotrexate and prednisone. *Arthritis Rheum* 38: 608–613

78   Black RA, Rauch CT, Kozlosky CJ, Peschon JJ, Slack JL, Wolfson MF, Castner BJ, Stocking KL, Reddy P, Srinivasan S et al (1997) A metalloproteinase disintegrin that releases tumour necrosis factor-α from cells. *Nature* 385: 729–736

79   Semmler J, Wachtal H, Endres S (1993) The specific type IV phosphodiesterase inhibitor rolipram suppresses tumor necrosis factor-α production by human mononuclear cells. *Int J Immunopharmacol* 15: 409–413

80   Le C, Nicolson A, Morales A, Sewell K (1997) Suppression of collagen-induced arthritis through adenovirus-mediated transfer of a modified tumor necrosis factor α receptor gene. *Arthritis Rheum* 40: 1662–1669

Methotrexate as an alternative to classic immunosuppressive therapies

Carol A. Langford[1] and Gary S. Hoffman[2]

[1]Immunologic Diseases Section, Laboratory of Immunoregulation, National Institute of Allergy and Infectious Diseases, National Institutes of Health, Bethesda, MD 20892, USA;
[2]Department of Rheumatic and Immunologic Diseases, Cleveland Clinic Foundation, Cleveland, OH 44195, USA

Introduction

The primary systemic vasculitides are a heterogeneous group of disorders which are characterized by inflammation of the blood vessel wall which may lead to compromise of the lumen and ischemia or attenuation of the vessel wall, aneurysm formation, and possible hemorrhage. Although the pathophysiology of vasculitis is not well understood, support for an immunological mechanism has come in part from the effectiveness of immunosuppressive therapy in the management of many vasculitic diseases.

Glucocorticosteroids (CS) were the first immunosuppressive treatment applied to the treatment of vasculitis. For some entities, such as giant cell arteritis and Takayasu's arteritis, CS alone have historically formed the foundation of treatment. While they have proved largely efficacious in such settings, the chronic and often relapsing nature of these diseases places patients at risk of significant short- and long-term toxicity from CS treatment.

In other forms of vasculitis such as Wegener's granulomatosis, CS alone are ineffective at treating active major organ disease manifestations, in particular glomerulonephritis. Wegener's granulomatosis had a universally fatal outcome until the introduction of combined therapy with CS and cyclophosphamide (CYC) [1, 2]. Although this regimen brought about a dramatic improvement in patient outcome, with the opportunity for long-term follow-up, we have gained a greater appreciation of the potential long-term toxicity of CYC treatment. Of particular concern, transitional carcinoma of the bladder has been observed in 6% of patients treated with daily CYC and by Kaplan-Meier estimates may reach as high as 16% at 15 years after first beginning CYC [3]. For these reasons, alternative immunosuppressive regimens have been investigated with the hopes of providing a safer option for treatment that is efficacious and yet minimizes the potential for long-term toxicity. Among these alternatives, the cytotoxic agent with which there has been the greatest degree of experience has been methotrexate.

Disease-modifying Therapy in Vasculitides, edited by Cees G. M. Kallenberg and
Jan W. Cohen Tervaert

Historical background

Methotrexate (MTX) was first introduced in 1948 as an antineoplastic agent and it remains to this day the most widely used anti-metabolite for cancer chemotherapy [4]. During the 1960s, MTX began to be applied to the treatment of psoriasis. This remained a toxic treatment option for this disease until Weinstein and Frost, in 1971, reported on the use of low-dose weekly MTX which produced far less toxicity than daily therapy or larger dose parenteral injections [5]. During the 1980's, this regimen was extensively studied and used in patients with rheumatoid arthritis. From this long-term experience, much has been learned about the properties and side-effects of low-dose weekly MTX which has greatly aided its application to the vasculitides.

MTX is believed to have antineoplastic activity by inhibiting dihydrofolate reductase and interfering with DNA synthesis [4]. However, the mechanism of action of MTX in treating immune-mediated diseases remains unclear. MTX is thought to have a number of potential suppressive effects on both cellular and humoral immunity [6, 7]. In addition to its immunosuppressive properties, it has been postulated that MTX has anti-inflammatory activity that is related to its effects on adenosine metabolism. At pharmacologic concentrations, MTX has been found to increase adenosine accumulation and release from cultured fibroblasts and endothelial cells which in turn diminishes neutrophil adhesion to these cells [6, 7]. This has particular relevance to the treatment of vasculitis as neutrophil adhesion to endothelial cells may be an important step in the pathogenesis of these diseases.

The initial investigation of MTX as a therapeutic agent for vasculitis was supported by its theoretical mechanisms of action as well as encouraging results from early case reports. Prior to the first reported prospective studies with CYC and CS, MTX had been used to successfully treat a small number of patients with Wegener's granulomatosis [8–11] and polyarteritis nodosa [12–15]. Through this time, the experience with MTX in rheumatoid arthritis grew and beneficial results were also reported in individual patients who had cutaneous rheumatoid vasculitis [15–19]. With this background, standardized prospective trials were subsequently initiated to study the efficacy of MTX in vasculitis. The three forms of systemic vasculitis in which MTX has been investigated most extensively to date include Wegener's granulomatosis, Takayasu's arteritis, and giant cell (temporal) arteritis.

Wegener's granulomatosis

Wegener's granulomatosis (WG) is histologically characterized by the presence of necrosis, granulomatous inflammation, and vasculitis of the small to medium sized vessels. Although classicially viewed as predominantly affecting the organ triad of the upper airways, lungs, and kidneys, WG is a multisystem disease than can involve almost any organ. Untreated generalized WG runs a rapidly fatal course with a mean survival time of 5 months and a 93% mortality rate within 2 years [20]. Although CS alone have been found to delay mortality in some instances, they have not produced a sustained remission in patients with severe vasculitis [21]. The outcome for patients with WG dramatically improved with the introduction of treatment with daily CYC and CS [2, 22]. In 133 patients treated with this regimen, 91% of patients exhibited a marked improvement in their disease manifestations and 75% achieved a complete remission [1]. Despite this, disease relapse was found to occur in 50% of this population and 42% experienced serious morbidity as a result of treatment. For this reason, alternative regimens which are effective and less toxic have continued to be actively investigated.

MTX was first examined at the National Institutes of Health (NIH) for its ability to induce remission in selected patients with active WG who had non-life-threatening disease [23–25]. Patients were not eligible for this treatment if they had a serum creatinine > 2.5 mg/dl or pulmonary compromise with an arterial PO2 of < 70 mmHg, and/or carbon monoxide diffusing capacity < 70% of predicted. Other exclusion criteria included ongoing alcohol use, chronic liver disease, pregnancy, infection with the human immunodeficiency virus, or an increase in immunosuppressive therapy within 4 weeks prior to enrollment. In this treatment regimen, all patients initially received prednisone 1 mg/kg/day. This dose was continued for 1 month after which time if there was evidence of disease improvement it was tapered to an alternate day schedule and then discontinued. Oral MTX was begun concurrently with prednisone at an initial dose of 0.3 mg/kg/week not to exceed 15 mg/week. After 1 to 2 weeks this was increased by 2.5 mg each week up to a dose of 20–25 mg/week. In the absence of toxicity, this dose of MTX was maintained for 1 full year past remission after which time it was decreased by 2.5 mg each month and discontinued.

In this trial, 42 patients with WG were treated with MTX and CS. Although patients with rapidly progressive renal or pulmonary failure were excluded, 60% had active disease involving three or more organ systems and 50% had glomerulonephritis as defined by the presence of an active urinary sediment with red blood cell casts. Remission was induced in 33 of 42 patients (79%) at a median time of 4.2 months (Tab. 1). Of these 33 patients who achieved remission, 19 (58%) experienced a disease relapse at a median time to relapse of 29 months. The presence of glomerulonephritis at induction did not emerge as a risk factor for relapse. In 15 of 19 patients (79%), relapses occurred either after MTX was discontinued or after the dose had been lowered to less than or equal to 15 mg per week. Thirteen of the 19 patients who relapsed were treated with a second course of prednisone and MTX. Eleven (85%) achieved remission with the remaining two having smoldering disease. MTX and CS were ineffective at controlling disease activity in only three (7%) patients, who were then treated with CYC on which they achieved remission. Three fatalities occurred in this study, two from *Pneumocystis carinii* pneumonia and one

Table 1 - Clinical response in 42 patients with Wegener's granulomatosis treated with an induction regimen of methotrexate and prednisone

No. (%) surviving	39 (93)
No. (%) achieving remission	33 (79)
No. (%) with relapse after achieving remission	19 (58)
No. (%) that relapsed after 1 full year of remission	12 (63)
No. (%) off methotrexate at relapse	9 (47)
No. (%) on less than or equal to 15 mg at relapse	15 (79)
Median months to remission (range)	4 (1–17)
Median months to tapering to alternate-day prednisone	3
Median months to discontinuation of prednisone	7

Data from [24, 25].

from a pulmonary embolism. Transient toxicities that resolved with dosage reduction included elevated hepatic transaminase levels (24%), leukopenia (7%), and stomatitis (2%). Pneumonitis occurred in three patients (7%) and resolved without sequelae following drug discontinuation.

Since the publication of the NIH MTX trial, two other series have been reported using MTX for induction of remission in WG. In a series by DeGroot et al., 19 patients were treated with weekly intravenous MTX 0.3 mg/kg/week combined with low dose prednisone given at a median starting dose of 10 mg/day (range 5–50 mg/day) [26]. With this regimen, 10 patients (59%) achieved a complete or partial remission. Although fewer patients achieved remission in this series, it is possible that this was influenced by the relatively lower dose of CS used in their regimen. Significant side-effects, including opportunistic infections, did not occur. In a retrospective series of 19 patients treated by Stone et al., the combination of oral MTX and daily CS was found to effectively control disease with remission being achieved in 14 (74%) patients [27]. In their experience, the side-effect profile was extremely favorable, with fewer serious toxicities than those reported in the NIH series. Although a higher rate of relapse was observed, the interpretation of this is confounded by the absence of prospectively defined outcome measures.

The data from all of these reports provide support as to the effectiveness and comparative safety of using MTX and CS to induce remission in selected patients with WG who do not have life-threatening disease or who have a contraindication to CYC. With the exception of *P. carinii* pneumonia which can be prevented by prophylaxis, serious side-effects related to MTX have occurred infrequently and the overall risk of toxicity from MTX appears to be less than that from daily oral CYC. Unfortunately, disease relapse continues to be problematic. Given the favorable side-effect profile, investigations are ongoing to study the role of prolongation of MTX for 2 years after remission. As relapses have been observed to occur most frequently when patients were receiving less than or equal to 15 mg, the MTX dose should be maintained above 15 mg weekly unless precluded by hematological or hepatic function testing abnormalities.

MTX has also been investigated as a maintenance therapy once remission has been induced with CYC. Such an approach is attractive as it employs the use of CYC to achieve remission, but then uses the less toxic agent of MTX for remission maintenance. Another benefit of this regimen is that by using CYC for induction, it can be applied to all patients regardless of disease severity at presentation, provided they are then eligible to receive MTX at remission.

In a report by DeGroot et al., patients who received either intermittent pulse or daily CYC as induction therapy for WG were subsequently switched at partial or complete remission to intravenous MTX at a dose of 0.3 mg/kg/week for an unstandardized length of time with or without concomitant prednisone [28]. A partial or complete remission was maintained in 86% of the 22 patients who received MTX alone followed for a median of 16 months, and in 91% of the 11 patients who received MTX and prednisone followed for a median of 22 months. Adverse events were observed in 12 of 33 patients treated with MTX with the toxicities including nausea (18%), transient leukopenia (15%), stomatitis (9%), pneumonitis (3%).

In an open label, standardized trial at the NIH, the role of MTX for remission maintenance after CYC induction was prospectively examined [29]. In this regimen, patients received prednisone 1 mg/kg/day tapered along an alternate schedule together with CYC 2 mg/kg/day given all at once in the morning. During CYC therapy, leukopenia was deliberately avoided by obtaining a complete blood count every 1–2 weeks and adjusting the CYC dose downwards to maintain the total white blood count above 3000/mm^3 (or a neutrophil count above 1500/mm^3). Once remission was achieved, CYC was discontinued and MTX was given orally at a dose of 20–25 mg/week. This was continued for 2 years and then tapered and discontinued.

Thirty-one patients were entered into this study, of whom 17 (55%) had glomerulonephritis and 16 (52%) had severe disease defined by specific renal, pulmonary, or neurologic criteria. No patient deaths occurred during this study and remission was achieved in all 31 patients (100%) at a median time of 3 months (range 1–12 months) (Tab. 2). Disease relapse occurred in five (16%) patients, all of whom were on MTX alone at the time of relapse and had been off of prednisone a minimum of 6 months. Neither glomerulonephritis, nor the presence of severe disease was associated with relapse. The median follow-up time since remission of the 31 patients was 16 months (range 4–49 months). The toxicities observed during this study included MTX pneumonitis (6%), leukopenia (10%-CYC, 13%-MTX), cystitis (6%), non-infectious CS toxicities (10%), bacterial pneumonia (6%), herpes zoster (13%).

The results of this study support that patients with active WG can be safely and effectively treated with a regimen using CS and daily CYC to induce disease remis-

Table 2 - *Clinical response in 31 patients with Wegener's granulomatosis treated with a cyclophosphamide and glucocorticoid induction and methotrexate remission-maintenance regimen.*

Number (%) surviving	31 (100)
Number (%) achieving remission	31 (100)
Number (%) with relapse after achieving remission	5 (16)
Median months from remission to relapse in five patients (range)	13 (10–15)
Median months off prednisone before relapse occurred in five patients (range)	8 (6–10)
Median months to remission (range)	3 (1–12)
Median months to tapering to alternate-day prednisone (range)	4 (2–8)
Median months to discontinuation of prednisone	8 (5–21)

Data from [29]

sion, followed by weekly MTX for remission maintenance. This regimen appears to provide a less toxic alternative to the standard CYC regimen, and can be used in all patients eligible to receive MTX at remission, regardless of initial disease severity.

In summary, recent investigations with MTX have continued to expand the therapeutic options available to patients with WG. Although daily CYC combined with CS is the most effective treatment for active WG and should be used in any patient with immediately life-threatening disease, long-term use of this regimen can be associated with significant toxicity. For this reason, current therapeutic approaches have become increasingly based on regimens that address the severity of disease while minimizing the potential for long-term toxicity. Recent studies have suggested that in appropriate settings, MTX may be considered as an alternative to CYC either for the induction of non-immediately life-threatening disease or for the maintenance of remission in patients who have had remission successfully induced by CYC. In this manner, MTX has been found to be a useful medication in the therapeutic armamentarium for WG.

Takayasu's arteritis

Takayasu's arteritis (TA) is a systemic inflammatory disease that usually includes the aorta and/or its primary branches. It is a rare disease, estimated to occur in ~2.6 persons per million per year. Young Asian females are disproportionately represented in most series, however, TA is becoming increasingly recognized in Caucasians, persons of African ancestry, males and individuals greater than 40 years of age [30–34]. TA has often been viewed as a triphasic disease in which the onset is systemic and not vascular targeted, followed by a vascular inflammatory phase and then a burnt-out phase. However, long-term studies have questioned the simplicity of this concept as it ignores many in whom the course of disease is either one of recurrent episodes or chronic and persistent, with waxing and waning disease activity [30, 32]. The latter concept emphasizes that treatment includes a need for life-long surveillance. Mortality has been reported to range from as little as 3% to 35% in the first 5 years of disease [30, 35]. Morbidity from disease and treatment has been estimated to cause partial or complete disability in up to 75% of patients [30]. In spite of these sobering observations, current medical and surgical therapy, applied by experienced practitioners, has been successful in reducing morbidity and mortality in TA.

Among the most difficult management problems in TA is recognition and treatment of clinically silent progressive disease. Inflammatory markers such as clinical features, erythrocyte sedimentation rate (ESR), or von Willebrand factor antigen are not sufficiently sensitive or specific to identify all patients with active disease [30, 32, 36, 37]. Active disease in asymptomatic individuals has been recognized by periodic arteriographic studies, which have revealed new sites of stenosis or aneurysm formation. Still other individuals who are clinically "silent", but require bypass surgery for old critically stenotic lesions, may provide histopathologic evidence of unsuspected active disease from tissue obtained at the time of surgery [30, 36]. This inability to accurately assess disease activity has provided a critical limitation in evaluating therapeutic interventions both within the context of a clinical trial as well as in management of the individual patient.

The ideal goal of medical therapy to prevent permanent vascular morphologic changes is often not achieved and patients with TA may experience clinical deterioration as a result of non-inflammatory disease. Hypertension is one of the leading causes of morbidity and mortality in TA and contributes more often to cerebro-, cardio- and reno-vascular organ failure than primary vascular stenotic lesions. Whenever feasible, anatomic correction of aggravating or causative lesions (e.g. renal artery stenosis) should be attempted. In addition to the treatment of renal artery lesions, vascular bypass procedures have been successful in diminishing morbidity and mortality in carefully selected patients with cerebral, coronary, and peripheral ischemic vascular disease [38]. Less often dilatation of the aortic root may lead to severe aortic regurgitation, requiring an aortic graft and aortic valve replacement. The usual limitations of vascular surgery are further complicated by the possibility of active arteritis leading to occlusion at the graft origin or insertion. These observations emphasize the importance of intraoperative biopsies in all patients with TA undergoing vascular surgery [38]. The finding of unsuspected active disease obligates CS therapy. It has been assumed, although not proven, that the likelihood of sustained graft patency is enhanced by decreasing inflammation. Similar reasoning has been applied to recommendations for suppression of any suspicious signs of disease activity before surgery.

About 20% of patients with TA may have a monophasic and self-limiting illness that does not require immunosuppressive treatment. Most of these individuals are identified in the course of routine examinations at which pulse deficits, asymmetries or bruits are recognized. Subsequent vascular imaging studies may then reveal typical patterns of stenoses and or aneurysms of the aorta and its primary branches. Other patients are identified because of symptoms of extremity claudication, other ischemic events and constitutional symptoms. Many of these patients that have symptoms or serologic markers (e.g. elevated ESR) of active disease, readily respond to CS therapy and some may be successfully tapered off this agent without disease relapse. A 20-year study from the NIH revealed that 80% of their 60 patients presented with active disease and required treatment [30]. Therapy with prednisone 1 mg/kg/day, followed by slow tapering of dosage, lead to 60% of patients being able to achieve CS-free remissions. However, 50% of CS treated patients relapsed in the course of tapering drug or shortly after its discontinuation. Retreatment included a cytotoxic agent. Forty percent of those treated with a cytotoxic agent (CYC or MTX) and CS achieved remission, but in time about half of these patients relapsed as well. Twenty-three percent of all treated patients had continuous disease activity regardless of therapy [30, 32, 39].

Hoffman et al. performed a prospective standardized trial investigating the utility of MTX in TA in patients who failed to achieve remission with CS therapy alone or who relapsed shortly after tapering and discontinuation of CS [40]. In this protocol, patients initially received MTX 0.3 mg/kg/week, not to exceed 15 mg/week. The dose was then gradually increased by 2.5 mg every 1–2 weeks, up to a maximum dose of 25 mg/week. Prednisone was begun concurrently at 1 mg/kg/day, which was tapered after 1 month, with the goal of achieving an every other day regimen (60 mg every other day) within 3–6 months. The use of combined CS and MTX led to remissions in 81% of 16 patients. However, 44% again had relapses as CS were tapered to or were near discontinuation. Overall, 50% of patients sustained remissions that had not previously been possible. In 25% of the group, remissions were sustained in the absence of any therapy (mean follow-up = 11.3 months). *P. carinii* pneumonia occurred in one patient which was successfully treated. Other toxicities included elevated hepatic transaminase levels (28%), nausea (22%), and stomatitis (6%) all of which were eliminated by reduction in MTX dosage. The evidence from this study suggests that MTX is of value in patients with treatment-resistant TA.

Anecdotal reports of attempts to achieve remission with new agents, after conventional therapies have failed, emphasize the limitations of medical therapy for TA. In a recent study, mycophenolate mofetil appeared to produce substantial improvement in three patients who had failed more conventional therapies [41]. The role of this agent in TA will have to be determined in larger trials. It has become clear that the effectiveness of medical therapy is not as great as once believed. Major breakthroughs in the therapy of TA will require a much better understanding of disease etiology and pathogenesis than is currently available.

Giant cell arteritis

Giant cell arteritis (GCA) affects about one in 600 patients over the age of 50 years [42]. Apart from a positive temporal artery biopsy, the most specific features of GCA are (1) new onset of an atypical headache, (2) jaw (masseter muscle) claudication, (3) abnormalities of the temporal artery upon palpation [42, 43] and (4) amaurosis [44].

CS continue to be the most effective therapy for GCA. Prednisone ~0.7–1 mg/kg/day will reduce symptoms within one to two days and often eliminate symptoms within a week. One month after clinical and laboratory parameters, particularly the ESR, have normalized, CS tapering is usually begun. Unfortunately the ESR is not always abnormal at the time of diagnosis, nor does it always normalize with apparent disease control. Between 1.2–20% of patients with biopsy proven GCA have been reported to have ESR values of < 20–30 mm/h [45–47]. Therefore the ESR or other imperfect surrogate markers of disease activity should not be relied on as the sole parameter to guide modifications in therapy.

The dilemmas of treatment of GCA are further confounded by observations that patients may relapse as long as 10 or more years after successful therapy and discontinuance of treatment [48]. In addition, an uncertain number of patients thought to be in remission have unexpected findings of histologically active GCA at the time of surgery for aortic aneurysms or at the time of *post mortem* examinations, again raising questions about whether GCA in some or all patients is ever fully controlled or "burns out" [49, 50].

The morbidity of CS treatment for GCA can be profound. Rob-Nicholson et al. [51] noted a five-fold increase in fractures and a three-fold increase in cataracts in CS-treated patients compared to patients initially suspected, but not proven to have GCA, who were not treated (follow-up = 5 years). Other CS-related side-effects have been less carefully studied. They include Cushingoid habitus, new-onset diabetes mellitus, gastritis, peptic ulcer disease, hypertension, aggravation of heart disease, glaucoma, myopathy and opportunistic infections, to name but a few. Consequently, physicians who treat GCA and other forms of vasculitis have been committed to minimizing CS toxicity, while maintaining disease control. Different authors have reported a wide range in frequency of relapse in the course of tapering CS after initial improvement. This is no doubt in part related to marked variations in treatment protocols. Nonetheless, ~30–60% of patients can be expected to relapse during CS reduction or withdrawal [46, 52–54]. In addition, under the best of circumstances, occasional patients may either not achieve complete remission or not be able to be tapered off CS. Cytotoxic and other immunosuppressive agents have been recommended for such individuals by some authors, but the utility of these agents, as demonstrated by controlled trials, has not been adequately addressed [55].

MTX has been among the most commonly evaluated adjuncts to CS treatment for GCA. There is difficulty in interpreting and comparing results of different MTX studies because all suffer from at least one of the following limitations: (1) lack of a CS-only treatment group, (2) absence of blinding in study design, (3) small numbers of patients, (4) including both PMR and GCA within the study group or (5) having relatively brief follow-up periods. In addition, substantial differences in CS and/or MTX doses between studies preclude direct comparisons. In spite of these limitations, it is important to note that two randomized, double-blind controlled studies did not find MTX to be a useful adjunct to CS in GCA [56, 57].

Treatment toxicity

The side-effects that can occur with MTX are outlined in Table 3 [58, 59]. Because of its specific side-effects, MTX is contraindicated in patients with pre-existing liver disease or chronic severe pulmonary impairment. In addition, as the drug is eliminated by the kidneys, MTX should not be given to patients with renal insufficiency as increased drug levels can occur and result in acute bone marrow suppression [60].

Infection remains a major cause of morbidity and mortality in immunosuppressed patients. Treatment with CS and a cytotoxic agent broadly suppresses protective host factors and can predispose patients to the development of infection with bacterial and opportunistic pathogens [61, 62]. *P. carinii* pneumonia is a particularly important opportunistic infection in immunosuppressed WG patients and was the most frequent severe toxicity observed in the NIH MTX induction study [24]. Because of the high incidence of this infection, it has become our practice to provide prophylaxis with trimethoprim 160 mg/sulfamethoxazole 800 mg (T/S) three times a week to all non-sulfa allergic vasculitis patients who are on daily CS in addition to a cytotoxic agent. Although increased hematologic toxicity has not been observed in these patients who have received T/S at a lesser dose for *P. carinii* prophylaxis, T/S should not be given at a therapeutic dose (trimethoprim 160 mg/sulfamethoxazole 800 mg twice a day) to patients receiving MTX as pancytopenia has been reported to occur [63–68].

Adjunctive folate therapy is often used to mitigate some of the side-effects of MTX that may be influenced by folate depletion [69, 70]. Studies in rheumatoid arthritis suggest that folate replacement may lessen gastrointestinal symptoms, mucositis, and bone marrow suppression, but does not affect hepatotoxicity or pneumonitis. The most frequent replacement regimens include the use of folic acid 1 mg daily or calcium leukovorin 5–10 mg once a week given 24 h after MTX. Because leucovorin is a reduced folate that can bypass the metabolic block created by MTX, there have been concerns that it may negate drug effectiveness. A biologically active leucovorin dosage of up to half of the MTX dose has been administered without an apparent change in efficacy although exacerbations of rheumatoid arthritis have been observed when the folate to MTX ratio exceeded this level [70].

Table 3 - Methotrexate side-effect frequency and strategies for prevention and monitoring

Toxicity	Frequency	Prevention, monitoring, or treatment strategy
Nausea	2–50%	Split dose to two or three portions over a 24 h period Administer by subcutaneous or intramuscular injection Use of mild anti-emetic; folic or folinic acid may be helpful
Mucositis	5–30%	Folinic acid 5–10 mg once a week 24 h after methotrexate or folic acid 1 mg QD
Bone marrow suppression	5–30%	Monitor CBC weekly while adjusting dose every 4 weeks thereafter
Increased transaminase levels (Hepatic fibrosis)	10–70% (1%)	Contraindicated in hepatitis or past/ongoing heavy alcohol use Monitor liver function tests and albumin every 4 weeks Liver biopsy based on criteria established by the American College of Rheumatology for the use of methotrexate in rheumatoid arthritis
Pneumonitis	5–7%	Consider in patients with cough, fever, dyspnea and interstitial pulmonary infiltrates Must be differentiated from disease or infection If occurs: stop methotrexate, if severe prednisone 40–160 mg/day Methotrexate contraindicated in severe chronic pulmonary impairment
Infection	5–10%	Prophylaxis for *Pneumocysitis* pneumonia*
Teratogenicity	Yes	Contraception

*Trimethoprim 160 mg/sulfamethoxazole 800 mg three times weekly or trimethoprim 80 mg/sulfamethoxazole 400 mg daily. For sulfa allergic patients inhaled pentamidine 300 mg every 3–4 weeks or atovaquone suspension 1,500 mg daily may be used.

Conclusion

Over the last 10 years, MTX has become increasingly investigated as an alternative therapy to traditional immunosuppressive regimens in the treatment of systemic vasculitis. Although MTX remains a potent cytotoxic agent which has the potential to cause drug-induced morbidity and even mortality, the overall side-effect profile has compared favorably to other treatment options. By providing a less toxic therapeutic option, it is a valuable agent in the treatment of certain vasculitic diseases. Despite potential efficacy and relatively low toxicity of MTX, disease relapse continues to be a significant problem in most of the vasculitides. Further investigations are needed to explore new ways of using currently available agents as well as developing new therapeutic modalities.

References

1   Hoffman GS, Kerr GS, Leavitt RY, Hallahan CW, Lebovics RS, Travis WD, Rottem M, Fauci AS (1992) Wegener granulomatosis: an analysis of 158 patients. *Ann Intern Med* 116: 488–494

2   Fauci A, Haynes B, Katz P, Wolff S (1983) Wegener's granulomatosis: Prospective clinical and therapeutic experience with 85 patients for 21 years. *Ann Intern Med* 98: 76–85

3   Talar-Williams C, Hijazi YM, Walther MM, Linehan WM, Hallahan CW, Lubensky I, Kerr GS, Hoffman GS, Fauci AS, Sneller MC (1996) Cyclophosphamide-induced cystitis and bladder cancer in patients with Wegener granulomatosis. *Ann Intern Med* 124: 477–484

4   Jolivet J, Cowan KH, Curt GA, Clendeninn NJ, Chabner BA (1983) The pharmacology and clinical use of methotrexate. *N Engl J Med* 309: 1094–1104

5   Weinstein GD, Frost P (1971) Methotrexate for psoriasis. A new therapeutic schedule. *Arch Dermatol* 103: 33–38

6   Cronstein BN (1995) A novel approach to the development of anti-inflammatory agents: adenosine release at inflamed sites. *J Investig Med* 43: 50–57

7   Cronstein BN (1996) Molecular therapeutics. Methotrexate and its mechanism of action. *Arthritis Rheum* 39: 1951–1960

8   Choy DSJ, Gould WJ, Gearhart RP (1969) Remission in Wegener's granulomatosis treated with steroids and azathioprine. *NY State J Med* 69: 1205–1209

9   Appel GB, Gee B, Kashgarian M, Hayslett JP (1981) Wegener's granulomatosis – clinical-pathologic correlations and long- term course. *Am J Kidney Dis* 1: 27–37

10 Weiner SR, Paulus HE (1989) Treatment of Wegener's granulomatosis. *Semin Respir Med* 10: 156–161

11 Capizzi RL, Bertino JR (1971) Methotrexate therapy of Wegener's granulomatosis. *Ann Intern Med* 74: 74–79

12 Tannenbaum H (1980) Combined therapy with methotrexate and prednisone in polyarteritis nodosa. *Can Med Assoc J* 123: 893–894

13 Fraga A, Mintz G, Orozco JH (1974) Immunosuppressive therapy in connective tissue disease other than rheumatoid arthritis. *J Rheumatol* 1: 374–391

14 Leib ES, Restino C, Paulus HE (1979) Immunosuppressive and corticosteroid therapy of polyarteritis nodosa. *Am J Med* 67: 941–947

15 Mitchell MS, Gifford RH, Bertino JR, Kenney JD, Malawista SW (1976) The treatment of disseminated vasculitis with methotrexate. *Inflammation* 1: 285–295

16 Espinoza LR, Espinoza CG, Vasey FB, Germain BF (1986) Oral methotrexate for chronic rheumatoid arthritis ulcerations. *J Am Acad Dermatol* 15: 508–512

17 Tiliakos N (1985) Pulse methotrexate (MTX) therapy for intractable cutaneous ulcers. *Arthritis Rheum* 28 (Suppl): S37

18 Upchurch KS, Heller K, Bress NM (1987) Low-dose methotrexate therapy for cutaneous vasculitis of rheumatoid arthritis. *J Am Acad Dermatol* 17: 355–359

19 Williams HC, Pembroke AC (1989) Methotrexate in the treatment of vasculitic cutaneous ulceration in rheumatoid arthritis. *JR Soc Med* 82: 763

20 Walton E (1958) Giant cell granuloma of the respiratory tract (Wegener's granulomatosis). *Brit Med J* 2: 265–270

21 Hollander D, Manning RT (1967) The use of alkylating agents in the treatment of Wegener's granulomatosis. *Ann Intern Med* 67: 393–398

22 Fauci A, Wolff S (1973) Wegener's granulomatosis: studies in eighteen patients and a review of the literature. *Medicine* 52: 535–561

23 Hoffman GS, Leavitt RY, Kerr GS, Fauci AS (1992) The treatment of Wegener's granulomatosis with glucocorticoids and methotrexate. *Arthritis Rheum* 35: 6112–6118

24 Sneller M, Hoffman G, Talar-Williams C, Kerr G, Hallahan C, Fauci A (1995) Analysis of 42 Wegener's granulomatosis patients treated with methotrexate and prednisone. *Arthritis Rheum* 38: 608–613

25 Langford CA, Sneller MC, Hoffman GS (1997) Methotrexate use in systemic vasculitis. *Rheum Dis Clin North Am* 23: 841–853

26 de Groot K, Muhler M, Reinhold-Keller E, Paulsen J, Gross WL (1998) Induction of remission in Wegener's granulomatosis with low dose methotrexate. *J Rheumatol* 25: 492–495

27 Stone JH, Tun W, Hellman DB (1999) Treatment of non-life threatening Wegener's granulomatosis with methotrexate and daily prednisone as the initial therapy of choice. *J Rheumatol* 26: 1134–1139

28 de Groot K, Reinhold-Keller E, Tatsis E, Paulsen J, Heller M, Nolle B, Gross WL (1996) Therapy for the maintenance of remission in sixty-five patients with generalized Wegener's granulomatosis. Methotrexate versus trimethoprim/sulfamethoxazole. *Arthritis Rheum* 39: 2052–2061

29 Langford CA, Talar-Williams C, Barron KS, Sneller MC (1999) A staged approach to the treatment of Wegener's granulomatosis: induction with glucocorticoids and daily

cyclophosphamide switching to methotrexate for remission maintenance. *Arthritis Rheum* 42: 2666–2673

30 Kerr GS, Hallahan CW, Giordano J, Leavitt RY, Fauci AS, Rottem M, Hoffman GS (1994) Takayasu arteritis. *Ann Intern Med* 120: 919–929

31 Hoffman GS (1996) Takayasu arteritis: lessons from the American National Institutes of Health experience. *Int J Cardiol* 54 (Suppl): S99–102

32 Hoffman GS (1995) Treatment of resistant Takayasu's arteritis. *Rheum Dis Clin North Am* 21: 73–80

33 Sharma BK, Sagar S, Singh AP, Suri S (1992) Takayasu arteritis in India. *Heart Vessels (Suppl)* 7: 37–43

34 Sharma BK, Siveski-Iliskovic N, Singal PK (1995) Takayasu arteritis may be underdiagnosed in North America. *Can J Cardiol* 11: 311–316

35 Morales E, Pineda C, Martinez-Lavin M (1991) Takayasu's arteritis in children. *J Rheumatol* 18: 1081–1084

36 Lagneau P, Michel JB, Vuong PN (1987) Surgical treatment of Takayasu's disease. *Ann Surg* 205: 157–166

37 Hoffman GS, Ahmed AE (1998) Surrogate markers of disease activity in patients with Takayasu arteritis. A preliminary report from The International Network for the Study of the Systemic Vasculitides (INSSYS). *Int J Cardiol* 66 (Suppl 1): S191–194; discussion S195

38 Giordano JM, Leavitt RY, Hoffman GS, Fauci AS (1991) Experience with surgical treatment for Takayasu's disease. *Surgery* 109: 252–258

39 Shelhamer JH, Volkman DJ, Parillo JE, Lawley TJ, Johnston MR, Fauci AS (1985) Takayasu's arteritis and its therapy. *Ann Intern Med* 103: 121–126

40 Hoffman GS, Leavitt RY, Kerr GS, Rottem M, Fauci AS (1991) Treatment of Takayasu's arteritis with methotrexate. *Arthritis Rheum.* 34: S74

41 Daina E, Schieppati A, Remuzzi G (1999) Mycophenolate mofetil for the treatment of Takayasu arteritis: report of three cases. *Ann Intern Med* 130: 422–426

42 Hunder GG (1997) Giant cell arteritis in polymyalgia rheumatica. *Am J Med* 102: 514–516

43 Gabriel SE, O'Fallon WM, Achkar AA, Lie JT, Hunder GG (1995) The use of clinical characteristics to predict the results of temporal artery biopsy among patients with suspected giant cell arteritis. *J Rheumatol* 22: 93–96

44 Rodriguez-Valverde V, Sarabia JM, Gonzalez-Gay MA, Figueroa M, Armona J, Blanco R, Fernandez-Sueiro JL, Martinez-Taboada VM (1997) Risk factors and predictive models of giant cell arteritis in polymyalgia rheumatica. *Am J Med* 102: 331–336

45 Myklebust G, Gran JT (1996) A prospective study of 287 patients with polymyalgia rheumatica and temporal arteritis: clinical and laboratory manifestations at onset of disease and at the time of diagnosis. *Br J Rheumatol* 35: 1161–1168

46 Kyle V, Hazleman BL (1989) Treatment of polymyalgia rheumatic and giant cell arteritis. I. Steroid regimens in the first two months. *Ann Rheum Dis* 48: 658–661

47   Ellis ME, Ralston S (1983) The ESR in the diagnosis and management of the polymyalgia rheumatica/giant cell arteritis syndrome. *Ann Rheum Dis* 42: 168–170

48   Graham E, Holland A, Avery A, Russell RW (1981) Prognosis in giant-cell arteritis. *Br Med J (Clin Res Ed)* 282: 269–271

49   Evans JM, O'Fallon WM, Hunder GG (1995) Increased incidence of aortic aneurysm and dissection in giant cell (temporal) arteritis. A population-based study. *Ann Intern Med* 122: 502–507

50   Lie JT (1995) Aortic and extracranial large vessel giant cell arteritis: a review of 72 cases with histopathologic documentation. *Semin Arthritis Rheum* 24: 422–431

51   Robb-Nicholson C, Chang RW, Anderson S, Roberts WN, Longtine J, Corson J, Larson M, George D, Green J, Bryant G et al (1988) Diagnostic value of the history and examination in giant cell arteritis: a clinical pathological study of 81 temporal artery biopsies. *J Rheumatol* 15: 1793–1796

52   Lundberg I, Hedfors E (1990) Restricted dose and duration of corticosteroid treatment in patients with polymyalgia rheumatica and temporal arteritis. *J Rheumatol* 17: 1340–1345

53   Delecoeuillerie G, Joly P, Cohen de Lara A, Paolaggi JB (1988) Polymyalgia rheumatica and temporal arteritis: a retrospective analysis of prognostic features and different corticosteroid regimens. *Ann Rheum Dis* 47: 733–739

54   Graham E, Holland A, Avery A, Russell RW (1981) Prognosis in giant-cell arteritis. *Br Med J* 282: 269–271

55   Wilke WS, Hoffman GS (1995) Treatment of corticosteroid-resistant giant cell arteritis. *Rheum Dis Clin North Am* 21: 59–71

56   Spiera RF, Mitnick H, Kupersmith MJ, Richmond M, Spiera H, Peterson M, Paget SA (1998) A prospective double-blind randomized, placebo-controlled trial of methotrexate combined with corticosteroids in the treatment of giant cell arteritis. *Arthritis Rheum* 41 (S): 520

57   van der Veen MJ, Dinant HJ, van Booma-Frankfort C, van Albada-Kuipers GA, Bijlsma JW (1996) Can methotrexate be used as a steroid sparing agent in the treatment of polymyalgia rheumatica and giant cell arteritis? *Ann Rheum Dis* 55: 218–223

58   Langford CA, Klippel JH, Balow JE, James SP, Sneller MC (1998) Use of cytotoxic agents and cyclosporine in the treatment of autoimmune disease. Part 2: Inflammatory bowel disease, systemic vasculitis, and therapeutic toxicity. *Ann Intern Med* 129: 49–58

59   Goodman TA, Polisson RP (1994) Methotrexate: adverse reactions and major toxicities. *Rheum Dis Clin North Am* 20: 513–528

60   Furst DE (1995) Practical clinical pharmacology and drug interactions of low-dose methotrexate therapy in rheumatoid arthritis. *Br J Rheumatol* 34 (Suppl 2): 20–25

61   Sneller MC (1998) Evaluation, treatment, and prophylaxis of infections complicating systemic vasculitis. *Curr Opin Rheumatol* 10: 38–44

62   Segal BH, Sneller MC (1997) Infectious complications of immunosuppressive therapy in patients with rheumatic diseases. *Rheum Dis Clin North Am* 23: 219–237

63 Govert JA, Patton S, Fine RL (1992) Pancytopenia from using trimethoprim and methotrexate. *Ann Intern Med* 117: 877–878

64 Groenendal H, Rampen FH (1990) Methotrexate and trimethoprim-sulphamethoxazole – a potentially hazardous combination. *Clin Exp Dermatol* 15: 358–360

65 Jeurissen ME, Boerbooms AM, van de Putte LB (1989) Pancytopenia and methotrexate with trimethoprim-sulfamethoxazole. *Ann Intern Med* 111: 261

66 Maricic M, Davis M, Gall EP (1986) Megaloblastic pancytopenia in a patient receiving concurrent methotrexate and trimethoprim-sulfamethoxazole treatment. *Arthritis Rheum* 29: 133–135

67 Thomas MH, Gutterman LA (1986) Methotrexate toxicity in a patient receiving trimethoprim- sulfamethoxazole. *J Rheumatol* 13: 440–441

68 Thomas DR, Dover JS, Camp RD (1987) Pancytopenia induced by the interaction between methotrexate and trimethoprim-sulfamethoxazole. *J Am Acad Dermatol* 17: 1055–1056

69 Shiroky JB (1997) The use of folates concomitantly with low-dose pulse methotrexate. *Rheum Dis Clin North Am* 23: 969–980

70 Morgan SL, Baggott JE, Vaughn WH, Austin JS, Veitch TA, Lee JY, Koopman WJ, Krumdieck CL, Alarcon GS (1994) Supplementation with folic acid during methotrexate therapy for rheumatoid arthritis. A double-blind, placebo-controlled trial. *Ann Intern Med* 121: 833–841

Intravenous immunoglobulin as immuno-modifying treatment

David Jayne

David Jayne, Department of Renal Medicine, Addenbrooke's Hospital,
Cambridge CB1 2SP, UK

Background

Although developed for the treatment of humoral immunodeficiency, pooled normal
human immunoglobulin suitable for intravenous use (IgIV) has a wide range of
immunoregulatory properties and has, since the early 1980s, excited interest as a
therapy for autoimmune disease. Attention has focused on the mechanisms of the
therapeutic effects of IgIV and the contribution an understanding of these mechanisms has made to knowledge of the immunopathogenesis of autoimmunity. There
has been widespread clinical use of IgIV as a second line treatment for many autoimmune diseases with relatively few randomised studies demonstrating its clinical
effectiveness.

Several factors have led to the investigation of a role for IgIV in the treatment of
vasculitis to improve on the inadequacies of current immunosuppressive treatments.
IgIV has been proven to reduce the incidence of coronary artery aneurysms in the
childhood vasculitis, Kawasaki disease [1]. The frequent association of primary systemic vasculitis with autoantibodies to neutrophil cytoplasmic antigens (ANCA)
confirmed the autoimmune basis for these vasculitides and provided a target for
immunomodifying therapy [2]. Lastly, infections or infectious agents are aetiological factors in certain vasculitides and can be neutralised by IgIV [3, 4].

Intravenous immunoglobulin

Intravenous immunoglobulin is prepared from over 10 thousand pooled plasma
donations using a multiple stage fractionation process [5]. Commercial products differ in the details of these stages, in the additives used to prevent autoaggregation of
IgG and to stabilise the preparation, and in their viral depletion or inactivation procedures. All products conform to a World Health Organisation standard, which
assesses IgG subclass distribution and antibody titre to certain microbial antigens

Disease-modifying Therapy in Vasculitides, edited by Cees G. M. Kallenberg and
Jan W. Cohen Tervaert

[6]. There is no direct evidence of differing therapeutic potential between products in autoimmune disease but the toxicity and safety of IgIV may depend in part on the preparative process.

Viral transmission and IgIV

Infusion of a blood product from a large donor pool necessarily raises concern over the risk of viral transmission [7]. Following epidemics of hepatitis C related to IgIV products, this risk has been minimised by optimising the fractionation process itself, which incidentally removes viral particles, by the screening of plasma donations for viral infection and by the introduction of specific viral removal stages, such as ultra-filtration, pepsin digestion or the use of detergents [8]. One patient with systemic vasculitis being studied for parvovirus B19 infection had a change in parvovirus genotype immediately following IgIV, which was attributed to viral contamination of the immunoglobulin [9]. More recently, the potential for the transmission of prions by blood products has led to further restrictions on donors and has contributed to a worldwide shortage of IgIV limiting the development of newer indications [10].

IgIV and autoimmune disease

Following initial observations in idiopathic thrombocytopaenic purpura (ITP) there has been extensive testing of IgIV across the spectrum of autoimmune disease [11]. The most convincing evidence for therapeutic improvement is in ITP, Kawasaki disease, dermatomyositis, Guillain-Barré syndrome and inflammatory bowel disease [1, 12–14]. Pathogenetic mechanisms differ between these and other IgIV responsive diseases, which has hindered the development of a unifying hypothesis to explain its effect.

The immunomodifying effects of intravenous immunoglobulins

Of necessity, studies exploring potential therapeutic mechanisms of IgIV have focused on individual aspects of the disease process. Their conclusions may not be generalisable to the effects of IgIV in the clinical setting or in other autoimmune diseases. Also, multiple mechanisms can be operative simultaneously; it is this multi-factorial property of IgIV that has frustrated a clear understanding of its immunomodifying potential. Early experience in ITP indicated a rapid effect in the majority of patients; subsequently demonstrated to result from blockade of Fc receptor clearance of autoantibody tagged platelets [11]. While the disease subsequently relapsed in some, others enjoyed long-term remissions.

These observations highlighted several aspects of use of IgIV in autoimmunity that recur across the field: firstly, the clinical response is variable between patients, particularly over the long-term [15]. Secondly, attempts have been made to interpret mechanisms of IgIV immunomodulation as being dependent on either the constant, Fc, region; or to result from binding of the variable, F(ab')2, region, implying certain antigenic specificities within the IgIV pool. Finally, mechanisms have been divided into immediate effects, for example, falls in inflammatory mediators, and later effects, such as the reduction in autoantibody secretion. The experimental evidence for immunoregulatory effects of IgIV and their relevance to vasculitis is discussed below (Tab. 1).

T cells

T-cell proliferation to alloantigens and T-cell cytotoxicity is reduced by IgIV *in vitro* [16]. This has been linked to the post-translational inhibition of interleukin (IL)-2 in the mixed lymphocyte reaction and to modulation of the production of many T-cell cytokines, including interferon γ (IFNγ) and tumor necrosis factor (TNF) by activated T cells [16, 17]. The inhibition is accompanied by a fall in IL-2-receptor production and an increase in IL-1 receptor antagonist activity [17]. In contrast, synthesis of the monokine IL-8 is significantly increased [17]. Similar results have been observed by studying cytokine mRNA levels from circulating mononuclear cells after IgIV infusion *in vivo*. Such non-specific actions on T-cell activity do not influence immune responses to exogenous antigens and have not been directly linked to reductions in T-cell autoreactivity.

T-cell subpopulations

The interaction between counter-regulatory T-cell subpopulations has been manipulated by IgIV to prevent disease in experimental encephalomyelitis, uveoretinitis and adjuvant arthritis by a switching from a predominant Th1 to a Th2 phenotype [18, 19]. These observations have been linked to clinical evidence of improvement following IgIV in the autoimmune T-cell disorders multiple sclerosis and birdshot retinopathy [20–22]. Patients with Guillain-Barré syndrome treated with IgIV have falls in TNF and IL-1 without changes in the Th2 regulatory cytokine, IL-10; however, elevated levels of IL-10 in Kawasaki disease fall rapidly after IgIV [23]. An opposing imbalance in favour of Th2 activity accompanies vasculitis and glomerulonephritis in the Brown-Norway rat after mercuric chloride [24]. IgIV reduced IgE and pathogenic autoantibody levels as well as tissue injury, in terms of proteinuria and vasculitis, in this model, when administered before or at the time of mercury injection but had no effect once the disease was induced [25, 26]. A bias of the

Table 1 - Immunomodulatory mechanisms of intravenous immunoglobulin

Target for effect	Nature of effect	Evidence in vasculitis
T cell	Inhibition of cytokine release Release of cytokine antagonists Reversal of counter-regulatory sub-sets imbalance Inhibition of T-cell activity through binding to cell surface antigens	Brown-Norway rat model
B cell/Autoantibody	Reduction in autoantibody secretion Stimulation of natural antibody secretion Blockade of autoantibody binding	Falls in ANCA after IgIV Increase in IgM and natural antibody levels Inhibition of ANCA induced neutrophil IL-1 release
Cytokines	Inhibition of effect Inhibition of monocyte TNF secretion	Fall in CRP and anti-inflamma- tory effect in vasculitis?
Complement	Inhibition of complement-mediated injury	Henoch-Schonlein purpura?
Fc receptor	Increased Ig catabolism Blockade of autoantibody-mediated cytotoxicity	
Endothelial cell	Inhibition of TNF or IL-1 induced adhesion molecule expression Inhibition of leucocyte adhesion Reducution in thromboxane A2 and endothelin release	
Infectious agents	Neutralisation of superantigen-induced T-cell activation Control of viral infection	Kawasaki disease, Wegener's granulomatosis? Parvovirus B19?
Nerves Fas (CD95)	Promotes myelination Promotes apoptosis	Vasculitic neuropathy? Churg-Strauss angiitis?

cytokine repertoire away from a Th2 phenotype has been observed following incubation of IgIV with staphylococcal superantigen induced T-cell cytokine release, where IL-4 secretion was inhibited while IFNγ and TNF were unaffected [27]. Imbalances in T-cell subpopulations are less distinct in human vasculitis, although Churg-Strauss angiitis has features of a Th2 response and current evidence points to a Th1 phenotype in Wegener's granulomatosis [28]. There is normalisation of deranged circulating lymphocyte subsets after IgIV in Kawasaki disease, with increases in CD4+ and CD8+ T cells, and CD5+ B cells; consistent abnormalities of these subsets have not been found in other vasculitides [29].

T-cell surface antigens

IgIV contains antibodies reactive with various T-cell surface receptors, including CD4, CD5 and the MHC class I receptor [30–32]. Biological effects of these interactions include inhibition of the mixed lymphocyte reaction and of CD8+ T-cell-mediated cytotoxicity [31, 32]. Although they have proved difficult to isolate, autoreactive CD4+ T cells are strongly implicated in vasculitis and their depletion abrogates disease and lowers autoantibody levels [33, 34]. Firmer evidence supports the contribution of autoreactive CD8+ T cells to vascular injury in giant cell arteritis [35].

B cells and autoantibodies

Antibody production by lymphocytes is depressed *in vitro* through ligation by IgIV of the B-cell receptor and B-cell FcγRII receptors [36, 37]. This mechanism would also account for idiotypic suppression of B-cell activity by IgIV as such ligation induces anergy or apoptosis of activated B cells [37]. Experimental and clinical evidence from *in vivo* studies shows a different picture with increases in B-cell activity manifested by rises in both IgG and IgM antibody production and circulating IgM levels (Fig. 1) [38, 39]. The increase in antibody levels is accompanied by a bias in antibody repertoire towards non-pathogenic autoantibodies. These observations have been explained by idiotype network theory to represent stimulation by antibodies in IgIV of "natural antibody" activity [40]. Natural antibodies are proposed to have regulatory functions, through idiotype:anti-idiotype interactions, such as suppressing pathogenetic autoantibody production. The IgM fraction of normal plasma is enriched in natural antibody activity and the increase in total IgM seen in patients with vasculitis after IgIV has been linked with concurrent falls in ANCA levels (Fig. 2) [39].

Elegant experiments demonstrated a blocking effect of IgIV on autoantibodies in acquired anti-factor VIII disease which was dependent on the F(ab')2 rather than Fc

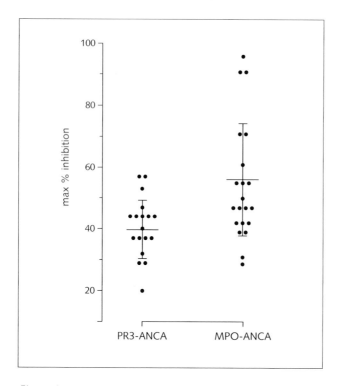

Figure 1
Inhibition of PR3-ANCA (n = 18) and MPO-ANCA (n = 20) binding by IgIV F(ab')2 frag-
ments (median ± SD) [91].

portion of IgIV [41]. This suggested binding of the variable region of IgIV molecules to idiotypes on the autoantibodies. Subsequent studies showed the same phenomenon in vasculitis: IgIV F(ab')2 fragments blocked the binding of ANCA to solid phase antigens, ANCA autoantibodies were preferentially adsorbed onto columns of immobilised IgIV, and in a reverse experiment, the ANCA inhibitory activity within IgIV could be enhanced by adsorption against ANCA rich immunoglobulin (Fig. 3) [42–44]. Inhibition of ANCA binding by IgIV was also found in the majority of a panel of 21 sera tested indicating the presence of a public idiotype on ANCA recognised by immunoglobulin from other individuals [42]. Functional effects of ANCA inhibition have been confirmed with the reduction in neutrophil IL-1 release *in vitro* [45].

An idiotype on PR3-ANCA, 5/7id, has been determined by a monoclonal antibody [46]. The 5/7 id is detectable in the immunoglobulin of 50% of patients with vasculitis and anti-5/7 id antibodies inhibit the binding of PR3-ANCA to PR3; how-

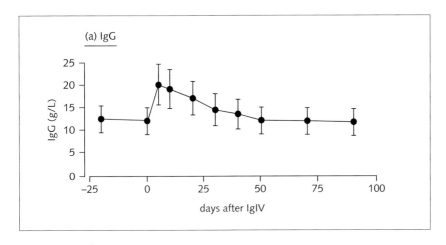

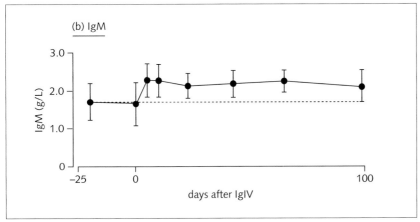

Figure 2
Changes in total IgG and IgM levels after IgIV infusion in systemic vasculitis [39].

ever, it is not known to what extent the 5/7 id is involved in IgIV-mediated interactions with ANCA [46]. A similar approach using the monoclonal antibody 7F2C11 has identified a common idiotype on MPO-ANCA, which also inhibits binding of MPO-ANCA to MPO [47]. This study additionally showed restricted clonotypes of MPO-ANCA using iso-electric focusing [47]. The apparent restriction in ANCA idiotypes would increase the frequency of idiotypic interactions between IgIV and ANCA and has raised the possibility of monoclonal anti-idiotypic therapy.

Post-recovery, ANCA-negative, sera also contains antibodies that inhibit ANCA and sequential studies have revealed an inverse relationship between levels of ANCA

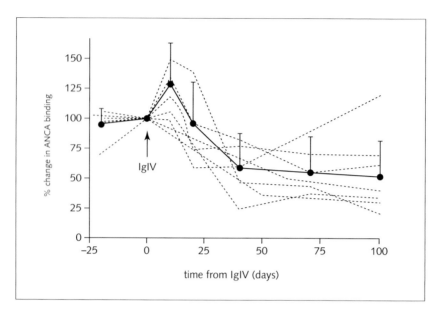

Figure 3
Change in ANCA level after IgIV infusion [88].

and ANCA anti-idiotype antibodies between active disease and remission [48]. Thus there appear to be public, common idiotypes on the majority of PR3 and MPO-ANCA which interact with physiological anti-idiotype antibodies present in normal and post-recovery sera. This evidence supports, but does not confirm, a role for idiotypic regulation in the control of ANCA expression that would be amenable to influence by IgIV. Most of these studies have involved the IgG fraction of sera, however preliminary evidence points to greater ANCA anti-idiotype activity in the IgM fraction. For example, the purified IgG from certain ANCA negative post-recovery sera has exhibited ANCA activity indicating a non-IgG factor preventing ANCA detection in whole sera [42].

Cytokines

The secretion of cytokines from peripheral mononuclear cells, including monocyte/macrophages is influenced by IgIV, but the pattern varies between the *in vitro* systems tested [17, 49]. The release of TNF and IL-1 by stimulated mononuclear cells is inhibited by IgIV and there is a selective increase in transcription and secretion of the IL-1 inhibitors IL-1ra and sIL-1rII and IL-8 [50, 51]. Circulating levels of TNF and IL-1 fall after IgIV in Guillain-Barre syndrome [52]. *In vivo* effects of IgIV in immunodeficiency have been contradictory with decreases in IL-1 activity in hypogammaglobulinaemia and increases in TNF and IL-2 in combined variable immune-deficiency when given in replacement doses, 0.2–0.4g/kg [51, 53]. The reduction in IL-1 activity following IgIV in Kawasaki disease appears to be related to anti-IL-1 antibodies in IgIV rather than a fall in IL-1 production [54].

IgIV contains immunoglobulin that binds to other cytokines and is capable of neutralising their biological effects, including TNF, GM-CSF, IFNα, IFNγ, IL-2 and IL-6, and leads to reduced anti-viral activity of post-IgIV sera [55–57]. Antibodies purified from IgIV have potent anti-IL-6 activity interfering both with binding of IL-6 to surface IL-6 receptors and with the formation of high affinity complexes mediated by IL-6 receptor beta chains [58]. Staphylococcal toxins are potent stimulators of monocyte TNF release and anti-toxin antibodies in IgIV reverse this effect [59]. The *in vivo* effects of IgIV on TNF induced inflammation has been studied in a hepatic microvascular model, where endothelial adhesion molecule expression and leucocyte adhesion was completely blocked [60]. Alternative mechanisms are also involved because the prevention of TNF-induced cytotoxicity by IgIV can occur after removal of TNF from the system, suggesting actions by IgIV on intracellular signalling [61].

Complement

Complement-mediated injury is abrogated by IgIV due to the absorption of activated complement fragments by antibodies in IgIV [62]. This mechanism appears to prevent endothelial complement deposition in dermatomyositis [13, 63]. The role of complement in vasculitides without immune complex deposition is controversial. However, sensitive techniques have detected the presence of activated complement and the C5–9 terminal attack complex on endothelium, polymorphisms of C3 are associated with the presence of vasculitis, and complement breakdown products promote neutrophil degranulation [64–66]. The interruption of complement activity through these mechanisms together with the impairment of complement's wider role in promoting immune responses are further candidate roles for IgIV in vasculitis [67].

Fc receptors

Monocyte phagocytosis *via* both FcγrI and FcγRII receptors is decreased by intact IgIV without major reductions in Fc receptor expression [68]. Fc receptor blockade explains the early rise in platelet levels following the use of IgIV in ITP, which has been reproduced by the use of Fc fragment infusions [11]. Fc receptor blockade by monoclonal antibodies impedes ANCA induced neutrophil activation, a process that may be mimicked by IgIV [45]. A newer proposed mechanism for reduction in autoantibody levels following IgIV is due to down regulation of the FcRn receptor. In health, this receptor recycles immunoglobulin from the intracellular compartment into the extracellular space; saturation of the receptor by IgIV promotes intracellular IgG catabolism hence reducing autoantibody levels [69]. This mechanism has not been thoroughly explored in autoimmune disease and does not explain continued reduction in autoantibody levels after levels of total IgG have returned to pre-IgIV concentrations.

Endothelial cell

The endothelium may be regarded as the target organ in vasculitis and changes in endothelial function contribute to leucocyte adhesion, thrombosis and distal infarction. The effect of IgIV on adhesion molecules and endothelial cytokine and chemokine expression was studied *in vitro* where it was demonstrated that intact immunoglobulin inhibited TNF and IL-1 induced adhesion molecule expression but did not influence basal levels of adhesion molecule, cytokine or chemokine mRNA [70]. These results help to explain the reduction in leucocyte-endothelial adhesion seen by *in vivo* microscopy in hepatic inflammation induced by endotoxin and are of potential significance to vasculitis [71]. IgIV also contains antibodies which disrupt intercellular adhesion through binding to β integrins [72]. The secretion of thromboxane A2 and endothelin by human umbilical vein endothelial cells is inhibited by IgIV F(ab')2 fragments without reducing prostacyclin release which would contribute to an anti-inflammatory and anti-thrombotic effect of IgIV [73]. Binding of IgIV to other endothelial receptors results in the blockade of thrombin induced calcium translocation and nitric oxide release [74].

Microbial infection and superantigens

Widespread T-cell stimulation by bacterial superantigens contributes to the pathogenesis of Kawasaki disease and has been proposed to explain the link between staphylococcal infection and vasculitis in Wegener's granulomatosis [3, 75, 76]. IgIV blocks T-cell proliferation, blast transformation and T-cell cytokine release induced by streptococcal superantigens and reverses the relative expansion of Vβ3+ and Vβ17+ bearing T cells induced by staphylococcal enterotoxin B [17, 77–79]. These effects have been attributed to antibodies in IgIV which compete with bacterial superantigens for binding to the T-cell receptor or directly neutralise circulating superantigens [59, 77, 78, 80]. Chronic infection with parvovirus B19 is linked with vasculitis and the improvement following IgIV has been accompanied by control of viral activity [4].

Other mechanisms

Non-pathogenic autoantibodies in IgIV promote myelination in models of multiple sclerosis after binding to oligodendrocyte surface receptors [19, 81]. Clinical responses in multiple sclerosis are detectable but objective evidence for re-myelination in humans is lacking. IgIV also inhibits microglial phagocytosis, through both F(ab')2 and Fc dependent mechanisms, and retards fibrosis [22, 82]. Nervous system involvement occurs in more than 20% of cases of systemic vasculitis and an intriguing observation of IgIV clinical studies has been the unexpected improvement in peripheral neuropathy [83, 84].

Apoptosis of lymphocytes and macrophages is promoted by anti-fas (CD95) activity in IgIV and this activity is greatly enhanced by affinity-purification of IgIV against immobilised fas antigen [85]. This mechanism explains the actions of IgIV in toxic epidermal necrolysis where there is over-expression of CD95 on keratinocytes and is of interest due to the recent demonstration of impaired CD95 function in Churg-Strauss angiitis [86, 87]. Removal of autoreactive cells by apoptosis will contribute to resolution of autoimmunity but there is no evidence that IgIV influences this process *in vivo*.

Clinical studies

ANCA associated vasculitis

Initial experience with IgIV in Wegener's granulomatosis and microscopic polyangiitis used IgIV as an additional agent to standard immunosuppressive therapies in patients with poor disease control [43, 88–91]. Individual cases have shown dramatic clinical improvement, while others have not; response rates following IgIV in published series have varied from 40 to 75% [43, 91–93]. Studies have varied in the number of courses of IgIV and it is unclear whether multiple courses are effective where a single course has failed [43, 89]. Remissions have also been reported following IgIV in less common presentations, including recurrent thromboses in paediatric disease and central nervous system involvement, both in the context of Wegener's granulomatosis [94, 95].

The difficulty of divorcing the effect of IgIV from that of continuing immunosuppressive therapies prompted a prospective study of six cases where IgIV was used as sole therapy for untreated disease without threatened vital organ failure [96]. Four exhibited a sustained improvement in disease activity with falls in CRP and ANCA, two of whom relapsed after 1 year, while two had only a transient response (Fig. 4) [96]. More recently a double-blind, placebo-controlled trial of IgIV for persistent ANCA associated vasculitis has been completed [84]. Thirty-four patients with grumbling or relapsing disease despite conventional treatments

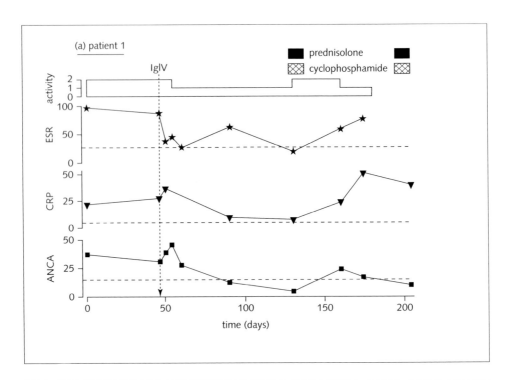

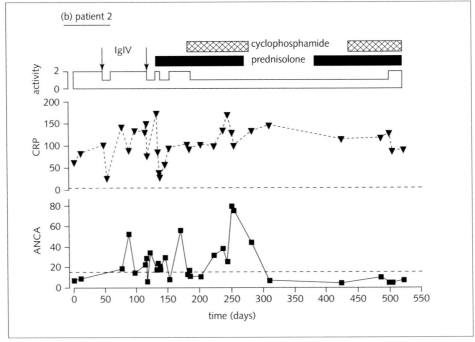

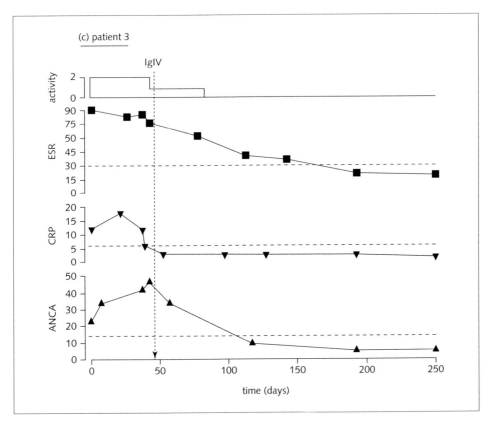

Figure 4 (left and above)
The treatment of ANCA associated vasculitis with IgIV alone. Three patients with differing patterns of response [96]. (Disease activity: 2, active disease; 1, partial remission; 0, remission; CRP, C-reactive protein).

received IgIV, 2 g/kg or placebo; the doses of immunosuppressive drugs were kept unchanged for 3 months at which time the primary end-point was a 50% reduction in the Birmingham Vasculitis Activity Score (BVAS) [97]. Fifteen of seventeen IgIV treated patients reached the end-point as compared to six of 17 in the placebo limb, and reductions in disease activity were mirrored by falls in CRP (Fig. 5), but were not sustained after 3 months [84]. Adverse-effects were frequent in the IgIV treated patients, with rises in serum creatinine of >20% occurring in four, aseptic meningitis in one and headaches with constitutional disturbance in seven. No differences in continued immunosuppressive exposure or relapse rate was seen after 3 months.

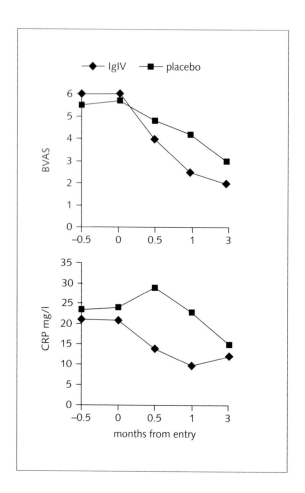

Figure 5
BVAS and CRP levels after IgIV or placebo in ANCA-associated vasculitis [84].

Circulating ANCA levels fall in some, but not all, patients after IgIV and have remained suppressed for at least 3 months [88, 89, 98]. The fall of ANCA *in vivo* has been compared to the *in vitro* ANCA-inhibitory activity of IgIV and to clinical responses; a preliminary study showed a correlation but confirmatory data is lacking [43, 84, 88].

The data above have led to protocols using intermittent IgIV at intervals of 3 months to maintain remission [99]. Five of the responder patients from the randomised study have continued on such a regimen with good effect [84]. Other IgIV responder patients have responded again when vasculitis has relapsed (Fig. 6) (D.R.W. Jayne, personal communication).

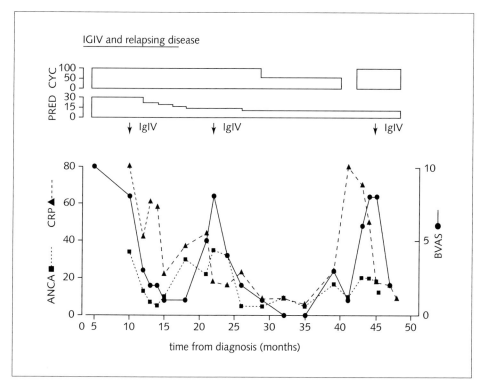

Figure 6
Repeated IgIV for relapsing ANCA-associated vasculitis. PRED, prednisolone mg/day, CYC, cyclophosphamide mg/day; CRP, C-reactive protein mg/l; BVAS, Birmingham Vasculitis Activity Score.

Churg-Strauss angiitis

A small number of case reports have demonstrated a therapeutic response to IgIV in Churg-Strauss angiitis [98, 100, 101]. This vasculitis is associated with eosinophilia, a feature of Th2 dominant immune responses analogous to that seen in the Brown-Norway rat model of vasculitis [26].

Henoch-Schönlein purpura

In contrast to primary systemic vasculitis, Henoch-Scönlein purpura (HSP) is associated with immune complex deposits that are related to dysregulation of IgA1 production and circulating IgA immune complexes. Two prospective studies involving 24 patients with IgA nephropathy (IgAN), the renal-limited variant of HSP, or HSP have found improvements in nephritis accompanied by reductions in IgA and β1 microglobulin levels, and glomerular IgA and C3 deposition following prolonged immunoglobulin therapy [102, 103]. The protocols used monthly IgIV, 2 g/kg for 3 months followed by intra-muscular IgG (IMIg), or IMIg alone for the less severe subgroup. Other, single case studies have reported improvements after IgIV in HSP with gut and renal involvement, and in steroid resistant HSP [104–106]. These results suggest an influence of exogenous IgG on IgA dysregulation in IgAN/HSP with consequent reductions in IgA mediated inflammation and injury. The nature of the interaction between therapeutic IgG and IgA production is not known but may be similar to that found in systemic lupus erythematosus where reduced immune complex deposition has been found after IgIV [107].

Polyarteritis nodosa

Recurrent, cutaneous polyarteritis nodosa refractory to immunosuppression has been controlled by IgIV in case reports [108–110]. A further treatment resistant case exhibited improvement during monthly IgIV treatment but relapsed subsequently [92]. Single cases of primary angiitis of the central nervous system and hepatitis B associated polyarteritis nodosa have shown dramatic responses to IgIV [111]. Paediatric polyarteritis, which is related to streptococcal infection in some cases, has been controlled by IgIV after the failure of other treatments [112–114].

Cryoglobulinaemia

There is a theoretical risk of exacerbating cryoglobulinaemic vasculitis with IgIV supported by the observation of severe leukocytoclastic vasculitis and acute renal failure developing after IgIV [115, 116]. The sequential combination of IgIV after plasma exchange is potentially safer because the cryoglobulin level is reduced by physical removal; such a procedure has been used in five cases of cryoglobulinaemic vasculitis (DRW Jayne, personal communication). Two Hepatitis C positive cases refractory to IFNα had prolonged treatment free remissions (Fig. 7), while in three hepatitis C negative cases, one showed no response and two enjoyed a partial response with improvements in constitutional symptoms, and reductions in immunosuppressive medication and requirement for plasma exchange. Another patient with hepatitis C associated cryoglobulinaemia failed to respond to IgIV and colchicine [92].

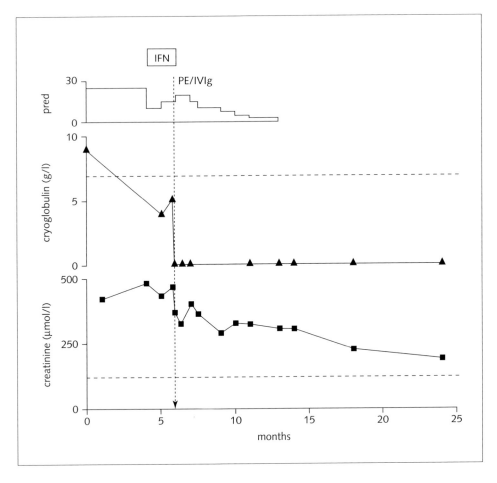

Figure 7
IgIV in hepatitis C positive cryoglobulinaemic vasculitis with glomerulonephritis.

Other vasculitides

Improvement in non-leucocytoclastic, ANCA-negative, severe skin vasculitis was found in 7/7 previously resistant cases with full remissions in five at a dose of 0.5 g/ kg every 4 weeks [117]. One from this series was withdrawn due to probable nephrotoxicity of IgIV. Further anecdotal reports attest to benefit with IgIV in chronic leukocytoclastic vasculitis and livedo vasculitis (atrophie blanche) [118, 119].

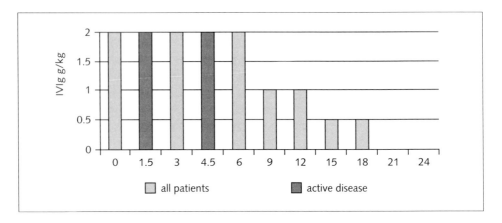

Figure 8
Consensus IgIV protocol for the addition of IgIV to conventional therapy in ANCA-associated vasculitis [99].

Administration of intravenous immunoglobulins

The dose of IgIV used in autoimmunity, typically 2 g/kg, has been higher than replacement doses for immunodeficiency, and approximates the size of the *in vivo* IgG pool. Dose ranging studies in Kawasaki disease have supported the 2 g/kg dose [120–122]. In ITP 1 g/kg is more effective than 0.5 g/kg [123]. Dosage frequency has varied from single courses for an acute indication to monthly or longer intervals. The European Study Group has developed a consensus protocol for the addition of IgIV to conventional therapy in new patients with ANCA-associated vasculitis, which awaits evaluation (Fig. 8) [99]. It has a tapering dose of IgIV at three monthly intervals and additional doses at 1.5 and 4.5 months for persistent disease. The clinical use of IgIV is limited by cost, at least US$ 20 per gram, and requires a cost benefit argument, as has been performed for IgIV in IgA nephropathy and HSP [124].

Toxicity

Nephrotoxicity

There have been over 100 reports of acute renal failure after high dose IgIV and it has become clear that this is not due to a hypersensitivity reaction but is a predictable result of administering large doses of immunoglobulin to patients with

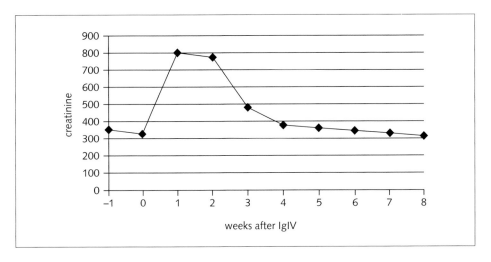

Figure 9
Acute renal failure after IgIV for systemic vasculitis in a patient with pre-existing renal impairment [84].

impaired renal function [84, 125, 126]. Many of the reports have involved products using sucrose as an additive to prevent aggregation of IgG prior to infusion, but it is not clear whether this bias is accounted for by the frequency by which these preparations are used. Sucrose is known historically to be nephrotoxic, causing very similar renal tubular abnormalities to those seen in renal biopsies performed after IgIV use [127]. However other factors may be important, including changes in plasma protein concentration and oncotic pressures after high dose IgIV or the presence of nephrotoxic IgG fragments filtered by the glomeruli.

In a placebo-controlled trial of a sucrose containing IgIV in vasculitis, four of 17 IgIV treated cases had marked rises in serum creatinine, observed in none of the placebo treated group (Fig. 9) [84]. Those manifesting a rise in creatinine all had baseline glomerular filtration rates below 40 ml/min. It is therefore probable that nephrotoxicity of IgIV is related to renal function and those with depressed function should either avoid IgIV or should receive lower doses over a longer period of time. Whether alternative or newer IgIV products are safer requires assessment.

IgIV and inflammation

Rises in ANCA were reported after IgIV using indirect immunofluorescence and these have been related to self-limiting flares in inflammatory activity [88, 93].

More serious inflammatory reactions, including vasculitis have been rarely report-ed [128–130]. Earlier ANCA assays used crude neutrophil extracts containing many antigens, and IgIV preparations have subsequently been shown to contain antibodies to such autoantigens, including bacterial permeability increasing protein and lysozyme which explains the apparent ANCA rise seen in previous studies [89]. Consequently, high dose IgIV infusion can lead to a "false positive" C-ANCA test although the pattern of fluorescence is usually atypical [131]. The presence of MPO-ANCA and PR3-ANCA was sought in 20 different batches of IgIV from one manufacturer and was undetectable in all (DRW Jayne, personal communication). Neutrophil activation leading to superoxide release can be caused by IgIV, and is inhibited by antibodies to FcγRII and FcγRIII [132]. This property is enriched in the dimeric fraction of IgIV and has been attributed to the binding of the Fc region [58]. The increase in IL-8 activity after IgIV is also pro-vasculitic as IL-8 is a potent inducer of neutrophil recruitment and antibodies to IL-8 abrogate experimental vasculitis [133].

Blood rheology

Blood viscosity rises sharply after IgIV particularly when given in high dose for immunoregulation [134]. Thrombotic complications of IgIV for these indications appear rare, with reported stroke and peripheral thrombosis in one case each, and myocardial infractions in four [135–137]. All had existing risk factors for vascular disease, and it would be reasonable to either reduce the IgIV dose or slow the rate of infusion together with offering anti-platelet drugs to such patients. Changes in blood viscosity may account for the retinal microinfarctions, which have been noted more frequently [93].

Future developments

The ANCA inhibitory activity of IgIV varies between IgIV batches and between manufacturers; selection of IgIV batches, or of plasma donors prior to IgIV purifi-cation has the potential to improve its efficacy in vasculitis [44]. The proportion of dimeric IgG is increased as the size of immunoglobulin pools increases and the dimeric fraction is enriched with self-reactive "natural" antibodies with high immunomodulatory potential [138]. This has been demonstrated after purification of the dimeric fraction in IgIV by size exclusion chromatography [139]. As discussed above, the IgM fraction of normal sera also contains variable region dependent inhibitory activity to ANCA and other autoantibodies [140]. The suppression of autoantibody activity by IgMIV is greater or equal to IgIV and also prevents exper-imental autoimmunity [141, 142]. Reductions in IFNγ and IFNγ-induced monocyte

TNF and IL-6 release were found with IgIV but not IgIV in one model [143]. IgMIV is also superior to IgIV in blocking complement activity [144].

The synchronisation of plasma exchange with IgIV has also been advocated to promote the immunoregulatory effects of IgIV [145]. Plasma exchange increases autoreactive B-cell activity and removes the diluting effect of the recipient's IgG pool [146]. Seven of 11 consecutive patients with severe autoimmunity responded to this procedure including one with Wegener's granulomatosis [145]. Further studies in vasculitis have combined immunoabsorption with IgIV [147].

Conclusions

The wide availability, relative safety and experience of IgIV in immunodeficiency have facilitated its testing in vasculitis. Also, academic interest in the immunoregulatory properties of IgIV, particularly idiotypic regulation, and the desire for non-immunosuppressive treatments in vasculitis, have provided a theoretical rationale. However, the lack of a clear understanding of the immunoregulatory activity of IgIV in vasculitis, its expense and the paucity of positive randomised trials have impeded its development as a routine therapy.

The immediate effects of IgIV are characterised by falls in CRP mediated by falls in inflammatory cytokines either as a direct action or indirectly by a reduction in lymphocyte and monocyte activity through Fc receptor binding, blocking complement or ANCA. Subsequent reductions of inflammation are likely to result from reduction in leucocyte/endothelial interaction, endothelial cell activation and complement deposition. The later fall in autoantibody levels, if it occurs, and maintenance of remission indicates control of B-cell and T-cell autoreactivity which can be explained by idiotypic regulation, restoration of physiological cytokine networks or abrogation of microbial superantigen stimulation.

Treatment of vasculitis with IgIV has not lead to sustained, drug free remissions in the majority of recipients but it has tended to be used in refractory or persistent disease where its evaluation is complex. However, the dramatic response in certain patients after IgIV and the insights IgIV might offer into immunoregulatory mechanisms has demanded further study. In particular, study of IgIV in autoimmunity has exposed novel mechanisms of cytokine and T-cell regulation by antibodies [15].

The existing clinical data makes a good case for further clinical trials of IgIV in vasculitis to assess efficacy in different subgroups of vasculitis and to determine the optimal dose and dose frequency. In particular, there is little data on its use in newly diagnosed patients where it may be most effective.

It is equally important to find factors predictive of a good response to IgIV and to start the evaluation of other immunoglobulin products, such as, IgMIV, the dimeric fraction of IgIV or IgIV prepared from plasma screened for anti-ANCA activity. Current immunosuppressive protocols have a high rate of adverse-effects of which infection is the most serious. IgIV offers the possibility of reducing immuno-suppressive doses while maintaining or improving therapeutic efficacy. This is particularly relevant to the elderly or pregnant patients in whom the adverse consequences of immunosuppression are more serious.

References

1   Newburger JW, Takahashi M, Burns JC et al (1986) The treatment of Kawasaki syndrome with intravenous gamma globulin. *N Engl J Med* 315 (6): 341–347

2   Hagen EC, Daha MR, Hermans J et al (1998) Diagnostic value of standardized assays for anti-neutrophil cytoplasmic antibodies in idiopathic systemic vasculitis. EC/BCR Project for ANCA Assay Standardization. *Kidney Int* 53 (3): 743–753

3   Cohen Tervaert JW, Popa ER, Bos NA (1999) The role of superantigens in vasculitis. *Curr Opin Rheumatol* 11 (1): 24–33

4   Finkel TH, Torok TJ, Ferguson PJ et al (1994) Chronic parvovirus B19 infection and systemic necrotising vasculitis: opportunistic infection or aetiological agent? *Lancet* 343 (8908): 1255–1258

5   Bos OJ, Sunye DG, Nieuweboer CE, van Engelenburg FA, Schuitemaker H, Over J (1998) Virus validation of pH 4-treated human immunoglobulin products produced by the Cohn fractionation process. *Biologicals* 26 (4): 267–276

6   Rutter GH (1994) Requirements for safety and quality of intravenous immunoglobulin G preparations. *J Neurol Neurosurg Psychiatry* 57 (Suppl): 2–5

7   Yap PL (1996) The viral safety of intravenous immune globulin. *Clin Exp Immunol* 104 (Suppl 1): 35–42

8   Dodd RY (1996) Infectious risk of plasma donations: relationship to safety of intravenous immune globulins. *Clin Exp Immunol* 104 (Suppl 1): 31–34

9   Erdman DD, Anderson BC, Torok TJ, Finkel TH, Anderson LJ (1997) Possible transmission of parvovirus B19 from intravenous immune globulin. *J Med Virol* 53 (3): 233–236

10 Milgrom H (1998) Shortage of intravenous immunoglobulin [editorial]. *Ann Allergy Asthma Immunol* 81 (2): 97–100

11 Imbach P, Morell A (1989) Idiopathic thrombocytopenic purpura (ITP): immunomodulation by intravenous immunoglobulin (IVIg). *Int Rev Immunol* 5 (2): 181–188

12 Hadden RD, Hughes RA (1999) Treatment of immune-mediated inflammatory neuropathies. *Curr Opin Neurol* 12 (5): 573–579

13 Dalakas MC, Illa I, Dambrosia JM et al (1993) A controlled trial of high-dose intravenous immune globulin infusions as treatment for dermatomyositis [see comments]. *N Engl J Med* 329 (27): 1993–2000

14 Levine DS, Fischer SH, Christie DL, Haggitt RC, Ochs HD (1992) Intravenous immunoglobulin therapy for active, extensive, and medically refractory idiopathic ulcerative or Crohn's colitis. *Am J Gastroenterol* 87 (1): 91–100

15 Kazatchkine M, Mouthon L, Kaveri SV (2000) Immunomodulatory effects of intravenous immunoglobulins. *Ann Med Interne (Paris)* 151 (Suppl 1): 1S13–1S18

16 Nachbaur D, Herold M, Eibl B et al (1997) A comparative study of the *in vitro* immunomodulatory activity of human intact immunoglobulin (7S IVIG), F (ab')2 fragments (5S IVIG) and Fc fragments. Evidence for post-transcriptional IL-2 modulation. *Immunology* 90 (2): 212–218

17 Andersson J, Skansen-Saphir U, Sparrelid E, Andersson U (1996) Intravenous immune globulin affects cytokine production in T lymphocytes and monocytes/macrophages. *Clin Exp Immunol* 104 (Suppl 1): 10–20

18 Pashov A, Bellon B, Kaveri SV, Kazatchkine MD (1997) A shift in encephalitogenic T cell cytokine pattern is associated with suppression of EAE by intravenous immunoglobulins (IVIg). *Mult Scler* 3 (2): 153–156

19 van Schaik IN, Vermeulen M, Brand A (1997) Immunomodulation and remyelination: two aspects of human polyclonal immunoglobulin treatment in immune mediated neuropathies? *Mult Scler* 3 (2): 98–104

20 Saoudi A, Hurez V, de Kozak Y et al (1993) Human immunoglobulin preparations for intravenous use prevent experimental autoimmune uveoretinitis. *Int Immunol* 5 (12): 1559–1567

21 LeHoang P, Cassoux N, George F, Kullmann N, Kazatchkine MD (2000) Intravenous immunoglobulin (IVIg) for the treatment of birdshot retinochoroidopathy. *Ocul Immunol Inflamm* 8 (1): 49–57

22 Achiron A, Miron S (2000) Intravenous immunoglobulins (IVIg) in the treatment of multiple sclerosis. *Ann Med Interne (Paris)* 151 (Suppl 1): 1S41–1S44

23 Noh GW, Lee WG, Lee W, Lee K (1998) Effects of intravenous immunoglobulin on plasma interleukin-10 levels in Kawasaki disease. *Immunol Lett* 62 (1): 19–24

24 Mathieson PW, Thiru S, Oliveira DB (1992) Mercuric chloride-treated brown Norway rats develop widespread tissue injury including necrotizing vasculitis. *Lab Invest* 67 (1): 121–912

25 Rossi F, Bellon B, Vial MC, Druet P, Kazatchkine MD (1991) Beneficial effect of human therapeutic intravenous immunoglobulins (IVIg) in mercuric-chloride-induced autoimmune disease of Brown-Norway rats. *Clin Exp Immunol* 84 (1): 129–133

26 Qasim FJ, Mathieson PW, Thiru S, Oliveira DB, Lockwood CM (1993) Further characterization of an animal model of systemic vasculitis. *Adv Exp Med Biol* 336: 133–137

27 Campbell DE, Georgiou GM, Kemp AS (1999) Pooled human immunoglobulin inhibits IL-4 but not IFN-gamma or TNF-alpha secretion following *in vitro* stimulation of mononuclear cells with Staphylococcal superantigen. *Cytokine* 11 (5): 359–365

28 Csernok E, Trabandt A, Muller A et al (1999) Cytokine profiles in Wegener's granulomatosis: predominance of type 1 (Th1) in the granulomatous inflammation. *Arthritis Rheum* 42 (4): 742–750

29 Lee HK, Kim DS, Noh GW, Lee KY (1996) Effects of intravenous immune globulin on the peripheral lymphocyte phenotypes in Kawasaki disease. *Yonsei Med J* 37 (5): 357–363

30   Vassilev T, Gelin C, Kaveri SV, Zilber MT, Boumsell L, Kazatchkine MD (1993) Anti-bodies to the CD5 molecule in normal human immunoglobulins for therapeutic use (intravenous immunoglobulins, IVIg). *Clin Exp Immunol* 92 (3): 369–372

31   Hurez V, Kaveri SV, Mouhoub A et al (1994) Anti-CD4 activity of normal human immunoglobulin G for therapeutic use. (Intravenous immunoglobulin, IVIg). *Ther Immunol* 1 (5): 269–277

32   Kaveri S, Vassilev T, Hurez V et al (1996) Antibodies to a conserved region of HLA class I molecules, capable of modulating CD8 T cell-mediated function, are present in pooled normal immunoglobulin for therapeutic use. *J Clin Invest* 97 (3): 865–869

33   Mathieson PW, Oliveira DB (1995) The role of cellular immunity in systemic vasculitis. *Clin Exp Immunol* 100 (2): 183–185

34   Lockwood CM (1998) Refractory Wegener's granulomatosis: a model for shorter immunotherapy of autoimmune diseases. *JR Coll Physicians Lond* 32 (5): 473–478

35   Brack A, Geisler A, Martinez-Taboada VM, Younge BR, Goronzy JJ, Weyand CM (1997) Giant cell vasculitis is a T cell-dependent disease. *Mol Med* 3 (8): 530–543

36   Kondo N, Kasahara K, Kameyama T et al (1994) Intravenous immunoglobulins suppress immunoglobulin productions by suppressing Ca (2+)-dependent signal transduction through Fc gamma receptors in B lymphocytes. *Scand J Immunol* 40 (1): 37–42

37   Spellberg B (1999) Mechanism of intravenous immune globulin therapy [letter comment]. *N Engl J Med* 341 (1): 57–58

38   Sundblad A, Huetz F, Portnoi D, Coutinho A (1991) Stimulation of B and T cells by *in vivo* high dose immunoglobulin administration in normal mice. *J Autoimmun* 4 (2): 325–339

39   Jayne DRW, Lockwood CM (1991) Stimulation of autoantibodies by intravenous immunoglobulin in patients with systemic vasculitis. *J Am Soc Nephrol* 2 (3): 596

40   Coutinho A (1995) The network theory: 21 years later [editorial]. *Scand J Immunol* 42 (1): 3–8

41   Sultan Y, Kazatchkine MD, Maisonneuve P, Nydegger UE (1984) Anti-idiotypic suppression of autoantibodies to factor VIII (antihaemophilic factor) by high-dose intravenous gammaglobulin. *Lancet* 2 (8406): 765–768

42   Rossi F, Jayne DR, Lockwood CM, Kazatchkine MD (1991) Anti-idiotypes against anti-neutrophil cytoplasmic antigen autoantibodies in normal human polyspecific IgG for therapeutic use and in the remission sera of patients with systemic vasculitis. *Clin Exp Immunol* 83 (2): 298–303

43   Richter C, Schnabel A, Csernok E, De Groot K, Reinhold-Keller E, Gross WL (1995) Treatment of anti-neutrophil cytoplasmic antibody (ANCA)-associated systemic vasculitis with high-dose intravenous immunoglobulin. *Clin Exp Immunol* 101 (1): 2–7

44   Pall AA, Varagunam M, Adu D et al (1994) Anti-idiotypic activity against anti-myeloperoxidase antibodies in pooled human immunoglobulin. *Clin Exp Immunol* 95 (2): 257–262

45   Brooks CJ, King WJ, Radford DJ, Adu D, McGrath M, Savage CO (1996) IL-1 beta production by human polymorphonuclear leucocytes stimulated by anti-neutrophil

cytoplasmic autoantibodies: relevance to systemic vasculitis. *Clin Exp Immunol* 106 (2): 273–279

46   Strunz HP, Csernok E, Gross WL (1997) Incidence and disease associations of a pro-teinase 3-antineutrophil cytoplasmic antibody idiotype (5/7 Id) whose antiidiotype inhibits proteinase 3-antineutrophil cytoplasmic antibody antigen binding activity. *Arthritis Rheum* 40 (1): 135–142

47   Nachman PH, Reisner HM, Yang JJ, Jennette JC, Falk RJ (1996) Shared idiotypy among patients with myeloperoxidase-anti-neutrophil cytoplasmic autoantibody associated glomerulonephritis and vasculitis. *Lab Invest* 74 (2): 519–527

48   Jayne DR, Esnault VL, Lockwood CM (1993) Anti-idiotype antibodies to anti-myeloperoxidase autoantibodies in patients with systemic vasculitis. *J Autoimmun* 6 (2): 221–226

49   Suzuki H, Uemura S, Tone S et al (1996) Effects of immunoglobulin and gamma-inter-feron on the production of tumour necrosis factor-alpha and interleukin-1 beta by peripheral blood monocytes in the acute phase of Kawasaki disease. *Eur J Pediatr* 155 (4): 291–296

50   Ruiz de Souza V, Carreno MP, Kaveri SV et al (1995) Selective induction of interleukin-1 receptor antagonist and interleukin-8 in human monocytes by normal polyspecific IgG (intravenous immunoglobulin). *Eur J Immunol* 25 (5): 1267–1273

51   Aukrust P, Muller F, Svenson M, Nordoy I, Bendtzen K, Froland SS (1999) Administra-tion of intravenous immunoglobulin (IVIG) *in vivo*-down-regulatory effects on the IL-1 system. *Clin Exp Immunol* 115 (1): 136–143

52   Sharief MK, Ingram DA, Swash M, Thompson EJ (1999) I.v. immunoglobulin reduces circulating proinflammatory cytokines in Guillain-Barre syndrome. *Neurology* 52 (9): 1833–1838

53   Sewell WA, North ME, Cambronero R, Webster AD, Farrant J (1999) *In vivo* modula-tion of cytokine synthesis by intravenous immunoglobulin. *Clin Exp Immunol* 116 (3): 509–515

54   Okitsu-Negishi S, Furusawa S, Kawa Y et al (1994) Suppressive effect of intravenous immunoglobulins on the activity of interleukin-1. *Immunol Res* 13 (1): 49–55

55   Menezes MC, Benard G, Sato MN, Hong MA, Duarte AJ (1997) *In vitro* inhibitory activity of tumor necrosis factor alpha and interleukin-2 of human immunoglobulin preparations. *Int Arch Allergy Immunol* 114 (4): 323–328

56   Ross C, Svenson M, Nielsen H, Lundsgaard C, Hansen MB, Bendtzen K (1997) Increased *in vivo* antibody activity against interferon alpha, interleukin-1alpha, and interleukin-6 after high-dose Ig therapy. *Blood* 90 (6): 2376–2380

57   Wadhwa M, Meager A, Dilger P et al (2000) Neutralizing antibodies to granulocyte-macrophage colony-stimulating factor, interleukin-1alpha and interferon-alpha but not other cytokines in human immunoglobulin preparations. *Immunology* 99 (1): 113–123

58   Teeling JL, De Groot ER, Eerenberg AJ et al (1998) Human intravenous immunoglob-ulin (IVIG) preparations degranulate human neutrophils *in vitro*. *Clin Exp Immunol* 114 (2): 264–270

59 Darville T, Milligan LB, Laffoon KK (1997) Intravenous immunoglobulin inhibits staphylococcal toxin-induced human mononuclear phagocyte tumor necrosis factor alpha production. *Infect Immun* 65 (2): 366–372

60 Ito Y, Lukita-Atmadja W, Machen NW, Baker GL, McCuskey RS (1999) Effect of intravenous immunoglobulin G on the TNFalpha-mediated hepatic microvascular inflammatory response. *Shock* 11 (4): 291–295

61 Stangel M, Schumacher HC, Ruprecht K, Boegner F, Marx P (1997) Immunoglobulins for intravenous use inhibit TNF alpha cytotoxicity *in vitro*. *Immunol Invest* 26 (5–7): 569–578

62 Basta M, Fries LF, Frank MM (1991) High doses of intravenous Ig inhibit *in vitro* uptake of C4 fragments onto sensitized erythrocytes. *Blood* 77 (2): 376–380

63 Basta M, Dalakas MC (1994) High-dose intravenous immunoglobulin exerts its beneficial effect in patients with dermatomyositis by blocking endomysial deposition of activated complement fragments. *J Clin Invest* 94 (5): 1729–1735

64 Dauchel H, Joly P, Delpech A et al (1993) Local and systemic activation of the whole complement cascade in human leukocytoclastic cutaneous vasculitis C3d,g and terminal complement complex as sensitive markers. *Clin Exp Immunol* 92 (2): 274–283

65 Finn JE, Zhang L, Agrawal S, Jayne DR, Oliveira DB, Mathieson PW (1994) Molecular analysis of C3 allotypes in patients with systemic vasculitis. *Nephrol Dial Transplant* 9 (11): 1564–1567

66 Tanaka T, Abe M, Mitsuyama T, Fukuoka Y, Sakurada T, Hara N (1995) Hyperresponsiveness of granulocytes to anaphylatoxins, C5a and C3a, in Churg-Strauss syndrome. *Intern Med* 34 (10): 1005–1008

67 Fearon DT (1998) The complement system and adaptive immunity. *Semin Immunol* 10 (5): 355–361

68 Jungi TW, Brcic M, Kuhnert P, Spycher MO, Li F, Nydegger UE (1990) Effect of IgG for intravenous use on Fc receptor-mediated phagocytosis by human monocytes. *Clin Exp Immunol* 82 (1): 163–169

69 Yu Z, Lennon VA (1999) Mechanism of intravenous immune globulin therapy in antibody-mediated autoimmune diseases. *N Engl J Med* 340 (3): 227–228

70 Xu C, Poirier B, Van Huyen JP et al (1998) Modulation of endothelial cell function by normal polyspecific human intravenous immunoglobulins: a possible mechanism of action in vascular diseases. *Am J Pathol* 153 (4): 1257–1266

71 McCuskey RS, Nishida J, McDonnell D, Baker GL, Urbaschek R, Urbaschek B (1996) Effect of immunoglobulin G on the hepatic microvascular inflammatory response during sepsis. *Shock* 5 (1): 28–33

72 Vassilev TL, Kazatchkine MD, Van Huyen JP et al (1999) Inhibition of cell adhesion by antibodies to Arg-Gly-Asp (RGD) in normal immunoglobulin for therapeutic use (intravenous immunoglobulin, IVIg). *Blood* 93 (11): 3624–3631

73 Oravec S, Ronda N, Carayon A, Milliez J, Kazatchkine MD, Hornych A (1995) Normal human polyspecific immunoglobulin G (intravenous immunoglobulin) modulates endothelial cell function *in vitro*. *Nephrol Dial Transplant* 10 (6): 796–800

74 Schussler O, Lantoine F, Devynck MA, Glotz D, David-Dufilho M (1996) Human immunoglobulins inhibit thrombin-induced Ca^{2+} movements and nitric oxide production in endothelial cells. *J Biol Chem* 271 (43): 26473–26476

75 Abe Y, Nakano S, Aita K, Sagishima M (1998) Streptococcal and staphylococcal superantigen-induced lymphocytic arteritis in a local type experimental model: comparison with acute vasculitis in the Arthus reaction. *J Lab Clin Med* 131 (1): 93–102

76 Hall M, Hoyt L, Ferrieri P, Schlievert PM, Jenson HB (1999) Kawasaki syndrome-like illness associated with infection caused by enterotoxin B-secreting *Staphylococcus aureus*. *Clin Infect Dis* 29 (3): 586–589

77 Takei S, Arora YK, Walker SM (1993) Intravenous immunoglobulin contains specific antibodies inhibitory to activation of T cells by staphylococcal toxin superantigens [see comment]. *J Clin Invest* 91 (2): 602–607

78 Baudet V, Hurez V, Lapeyre C, Kaveri SV, Kazatchkine MD (1996) Intravenous immunoglobulin (IVIg) modulates the expansion of V beta 3+ and V beta 17+ T cells induced by staphylococcal enterotoxin B superantigen *in vitro*. *Scand J Immunol* 43 (3): 277–282

79 Norrby-Teglund A, Low DE, McGeer A, Kotb M (1997) Superantigenic activity produced by group A streptococcal isolates is neutralized by plasma from IVIG-treated streptococcal toxic shock syndrome patients. *Adv Exp Med Biol* 418: 563–566

80 Takata Y, Seki S, Dobashi H et al (1998) Inhibition of IL-12 synthesis of peripheral blood mononuclear cells (PBMC) stimulated with a bacterial superantigen by pooled human immunoglobulin: implications for its effect on Kawasaki disease (KD). *Clin Exp Immunol* 114 (2): 311–319

81 Warrington AE, Asakura K, Bieber AJ et al (2000) Human monoclonal antibodies reactive to oligodendrocytes promote remyelination in a model of multiple sclerosis. *Proc Natl Acad Sci USA* 97 (12): 6820–6825

82 Stangel M, Joly E, Scolding NJ, Compston DA (2000) Normal polyclonal immunoglobulins ('IVIg') inhibit microglial phagocytosis *in vitro*. *J Neuroimmunol* 106 (1–2): 137–144

83 Nishino H, Rubino FA, DeRemee RA, Swanson JW, Parisi JE (1993) Neurological involvement in Wegener's granulomatosis: an analysis of 324 consecutive patients at the Mayo Clinic. *Ann Neurol* 33 (1): 4–9

84 Jayne DR, Chapel H, Adu D et al (2000) Intravenous immunoglobulin for ANCA-associated systemic vasculitis with persistent disease activity. *Qjm* 93 (7): 433–439

85 Prasad NK, Papoff G, Zeuner A et al (1998) Therapeutic preparations of normal polyspecific IgG (IVIg) induce apoptosis in human lymphocytes and monocytes: a novel mechanism of action of IVIg involving the Fas apoptotic pathway. *J Immunol* 161 (7): 3781–3790

86 Viard I, Wehrli P, Bullani R et al (1998) Inhibition of toxic epidermal necrolysis by blockade of CD95 with human intravenous immunoglobulin. *Science* 282 (5388): 490–493

87 Muschen M, Warskulat U, Perniok A et al (1999) Involvement of soluble CD95 in Churg-Strauss syndrome. *Am J Pathol* 155 (3): 915–925

88 Jayne DR, Davies MJ, Fox CJ, Black CM, Lockwood CM (1991) Treatment of systemic vasculitis with pooled intravenous immunoglobulin. *Lancet* 337 (8750): 1137–1139

89 Levy Y, Sherer Y, George J et al (1999) Serologic and clinical response to treatment of systemic vasculitis and associated autoimmune disease with intravenous immunoglobulin. *Int Arch Allergy Immunol* 119 (3): 231–238

90 Tuso P, Moudgil A, Hay J et al (1992) Treatment of antineutrophil cytoplasmic autoantibody-positive systemic vasculitis and glomerulonephritis with pooled intravenous gammaglobulin. *Am J Kidney Dis* 20 (5): 504–508

91 Jayne DR, Esnault VL, Lockwood CM (1993) ANCA anti-idiotype antibodies and the treatment of systemic vasculitis with intravenous immunoglobulin. *J Autoimmun* 6 (2): 207–219

92 Bahadoran P, De Bandt M, Echard M, Jarrousse B, Guillevin L (1993) Failure of intravenous immunoglobulins in certain systemic diseases. 5 cases. *Presse Med* 22 (25): 1175–1178

93 Blum M, Andrassy K, Adler D, Hartmann M, Volcker HE (1997) Early experience with intravenous immunoglobulin treatment in Wegener's granulomatosis with ocular involvement. *Graefes Arch Clin Exp Ophthalmol* 235 (9): 599–602

94 Adlakha A, Rao K, Adlakha K, Ryu JH (1995) A case of pediatric Wegener's granulomatosis with recurrent venous thromboses treated with intravenous immunoglobulin and laryngotracheoplasty. *Pediatr Pulmonol* 20 (4): 265–268

95 Taylor CT, Buring SM, Taylor KH (1999) Treatment of Wegener's granulomatosis with immune globulin: CNS involvement in an adolescent female. *Ann Pharmacother* 33 (10): 1055–1059

96 Jayne DR, Lockwood CM (1996) Intravenous immunoglobulin as sole therapy for systemic vasculitis. *Br J Rheumatol* 35 (11): 1150–1153

97 Luqmani RA, Exley AR, Kitas GD, Bacon PA (1997) Disease assessment and management of the vasculitides. *Baillieres Clin Rheumatol* 11 (2): 423–446

98 Levy Y, George J, Fabbrizzi F, Rotman P, Paz Y, Shoenfeld Y (1999) Marked improvement of Churg-Strauss vasculitis with intravenous gammaglobulins. *South Med J* 92 (4): 412–414

99 Jayne DR, Rasmussen N (1997) Treatment of antineutrophil cytoplasm autoantibody-associated systemic vasculitis: initiatives of the European Community Systemic Vasculitis Clinical Trials Study Group. *Mayo Clin Proc* 72 (8): 737–747

100 Hamilos DL, Christensen J (1991) Treatment of Churg-Strauss syndrome with high-dose intravenous immunoglobulin. *J Allergy Clin Immunol* 88 (5): 823–824

101 Armentia A, Fernandez A, Sanchez P et al (1993) Asthma and vasculitis. Response to intravenous immunoglobulins. *Allergol Immunopathol (Madr)* 21 (2): 47–52

102 Rostoker G, Desvaux-Belghiti D, Pilatte Y et al (1994) High-dose immunoglobulin therapy for severe IgA nephropathy and Henoch-Schonlein purpura. *Ann Intern Med* 120 (6): 476–484

103 Rostoker G, Desvaux-Belghiti D, Pilatte Y et al (1995) Immunomodulation with low-dose immunoglobulins for moderate IgA nephropathy and Henoch-Schonlein purpura. Preliminary results of a prospective uncontrolled trial. *Nephron* 69 (3): 327–334

104 Hamidou MA, Pottier MA, Dupas B (1996) Intravenous immunoglobulin in Henoch-Schonlein purpura [letter]. *Ann Intern Med* 125 (12): 1013–1014

105 Heldrich FJ, Minkin S, Gatdula CL (1993) Intravenous immunoglobulin in Henoch-Schonlein purpura: a case study. *Md Med J* 42 (6): 577–579

106 Kusuda A, Migita K, Tsuboi M et al (1999) Successful treatment of adult-onset Henoch-Schonlein purpura nephritis with high-dose immunoglobulins. *Intern Med* 38 (4): 376–379

107 Lin CY, Hsu HC, Chiang H (1989) Improvement of histological and immunological change in steroid and immunosuppressive drug-resistant lupus nephritis by high-dose intravenous gamma globulin. *Nephron* 53 (4): 303–310

108 Antonelli A, Agostini G, Agostini S (1992) Preliminary results of intravenous immunoglobulins in treating patients with vasculitis. *Clin Ter* 141 (9 Pt 2): 33–36

109 Uziel Y, Silverman ED (1998) Intravenous immunoglobulin therapy in a child with cutaneous polyarteritis nodosa [see comments]. *Clin Exp Rheumatol* 16 (2): 187–189

110 Machet L, Vincent O, Machet MC, Barruet K, Vaillant L, Lorette G (1995) Cutaneous periarteritis nodosa resistant to combined corticosteroids and immunosuppressive agents. Efficacy of treatment with intravenous immunoglobulins. *Ann Dermatol Venereol* 122 (11–12): 769–72

111 Boman S, Ballen JL, Seggev JS (1995) Dramatic responses to intravenous immunoglobulin in vasculitis. *J Intern Med* 238 (4): 375–377

112 Gedalia A, Sorensen R (1998) Intravenous immunoglobulin in childhood cutaneous polyarteritis nodosa [letter comment]. *Clin Exp Rheumatol* 16 (6): 767

113 Drymalski W, Hosen RS, Smook S (1994) Response to pooled gamma globulin therapy in a child with polyarteritis nodosa [letter]. *Arch Pediatr Adolesc Med* 148 (5): 543– 544

114 David J, Ansell BM, Woo P (1993) Polyarteritis nodosa associated with streptococcus. *Arch Dis Child* 69 (6): 685–688

115 Boom BW, Brand A, Bavinck JN, Eernisse JG, Daha MR, Vermeer BJ (1988) Severe leukocytoclastic vasculitis of the skin in a patient with essential mixed cryoglobulinemia treated with high-dose gamma-globulin intravenously. *Arch Dermatol* 124 (10): 1550–1553

116 Barton JC, Herrera GA, Galla JH, Bertoli LF, Work J, Koopman WJ (1987) Acute cryoglobulinemic renal failure after intravenous infusion of gamma globulin. *Am J Med* 82 (3 Spec No): 624–629

117 Altmeyer P, Seifarth D, Bacharach-Buhles M (1999) High dosage intravenous immunoglobulin (IVIG) therapy in therapy-refractory ANCA-negative, necrotizing vasculitis. *Hautarzt* 50 (12): 853–858

118 Ong CS, Benson EM (2000) Successful treatment of chronic leucocytoclastic vasculitis and persistent ulceration with intravenous immunoglobulin. *Br J Dermatol* 143 (2): 447–449

119 Amital H, Levy Y, Shoenfeld Y (2000) Use of intravenous immunoglobulin in livedo vasculitis. *Clin Exp Rheumatol* 18 (3): 404–406

120 Morikawa Y, Ohashi Y, Harada K et al (1994) A multicenter, randomized, controlled trial of intravenous gamma globulin therapy in children with acute Kawasaki disease. *Acta Paediatr Jpn* 36 (4): 347–354

121 Terai M, Shulman ST (1997) Prevalence of coronary artery abnormalities in Kawasaki disease is highly dependent on gamma globulin dose but independent of salicylate dose. *J Pediatr* 131 (6): 888–893

122 Newburger JW, Takahashi M, Beiser AS et al (1991) A single intravenous infusion of gamma globulin as compared with four infusions in the treatment of acute Kawasaki syndrome. *N Engl J Med* 324 (23): 1633–1639

123 Godeau B, Caulier MT, Decuypere L, Rose C, Schaeffer A, Bierling P (1999) Intravenous immunoglobulin for adults with autoimmune thrombocytopenic purpura: results of a randomized trial comparing 0.5 and 1 g/kg b.w. *Br J Haematol* 107 (4): 716–719

124 Durand-Zaleski I, Bastuji-Garin S, Zaleski S, Weil B, Rostoker G (1996) A cost analysis of the prevention of end-stage renal disease: immunoglobulin therapy for IgA nephropathy [see comments]. *Med Decis Making* 16 (4): 326–334

125 (1999) Renal insufficiency and failure associated with immune globulin intravenous therapy – United States, 1985–1998. *MMWR Morb Mortal Wkly Rep* 48 (24): 518–521

126 Blanco R, Gonzalez-Gay MA, Ibanez D, Sanchez-Andrade A, Gonzalez-Vela C (1997) Paradoxical and persistent renal impairment in Henoch-Schonlein purpura after high-dose immunoglobulin therapy. *Nephron* 76 (2): 247–248

127 Schifferli J, Leski M, Favre H, Imbach P, Nydegger U, Davies K (1991) High-dose intravenous IgG treatment and renal function. *Lancet* 337 (8739): 457–458

128 Ayliffe W, Haeney M, Roberts SC, Lavin M (1992) Uveitis after antineutrophil cytoplasmic antibody contamination of immunoglobulin replacement therapy. *Lancet* 339 (8792): 558–559

129 Hashkes PJ, Lovell DJ (1996) Vasculitis in systemic lupus erythematosus following intravenous immunoglobulin therapy. *Clin Exp Rheumatol* 14 (6): 673–675

130 Howse M, Bindoff L, Carmichael A (1998) Facial vasculitic rash associated with intravenous immunoglobulin. *Bmj* 317 (7168): 1291

131 Jolles S, Deacock S, Turnbull W et al (1999) Atypical C-ANCA following high dose intravenous immunoglobulin. *J Clin Pathol* 52 (3): 177–180

132 Nemes E, Teichman F, Roos D, Marodi L (2000) Activation of human granulocytes by intravenous immunoglobulin preparations is mediated by FcgammaRII and FcgammaRIII receptors. *Pediatr Res* 47 (3): 357–361

133 Qasim FJ, Mathieson PW, Sendo F, Thiru S, Oliveira DB (1996) Role of neutrophils in the pathogenesis of experimental vasculitis. *Am J Pathol* 149 (1): 81–89

134 Reinhart WH, Berchtold PE (1992) Effect of high-dose intravenous immunoglobulin therapy on blood rheology. *Lancet* 339 (8794): 662–664

135 Steg RE, Lefkowitz DM (1994) Cerebral infarction following intravenous immunoglobulin therapy for myasthenia gravis. *Neurology* 44 (6): 1180–1181

136 Go RS, Call TG (2000) Deep venous thrombosis of the arm after intravenous immunoglobulin infusion: case report and literature review of intravenous immunoglobulin-related thrombotic complications. *Mayo Clin Proc* 75 (1): 83–85

137 Elkayam O, Paran D, Milo R et al (2000) Acute myocardial infarction associated with high dose intravenous immunoglobulin infusion for autoimmune disorders. A study of four cases. *Ann Rheum Dis* 59 (1): 77–80

138 Tankersley DL, Preston MS, Finlayson JS (1988) Immunoglobulin G dimer: an idiotype-anti-idiotype complex. *Mol Immunol* 25 (1): 41–48

139 Vassilev TL, Bineva IL, Dietrich G, Kaveri SV, Kazatchkine MD (1995) Variable region-connected, dimeric fraction of intravenous immunoglobulin enriched in natural autoantibodies. *J Autoimmun* 8 (3): 405–413

140 Bar-Dayan Y, Bonnin E, Bloch M et al (2000) Neutralization of disease associated autoantibodies by an immunoglobulin M- and immunoglobulin A-enriched human intravenous immunoglobulin preparation. *Scand J Immunol* 51 (4): 408–414

141 Hurez V, Kazatchkine MD, Vassilev T et al (1997) Pooled normal human polyspecific IgM contains neutralizing anti-idiotypes to IgG autoantibodies of autoimmune patients and protects from experimental autoimmune disease. *Blood* 90 (10): 4004–4013

142 Vassilev T, Yamamoto M, Aissaoui A et al (1999) Normal human immunoglobulin suppresses experimental myasthenia gravis in SCID mice. *Eur J Immunol* 29 (8): 2436–2442

143 Nachbaur D, Herold M, Gachter A, Niederwieser D (1998) Modulation of alloimmune response *in vitro* by an IgM-enriched immunoglobulin preparation (Pentaglobin). *Immunology* 94 (2): 279–283

144 Rieben R, Roos A, Muizert Y, Tinguely C, Gerritsen AF, Daha MR (1999) Immunoglobulin M-enriched human intravenous immunoglobulin prevents complement activation *in vitro* and *in vivo* in a rat model of acute inflammation. *Blood* 93 (3): 942–951

145 Bussel A, Boulechfar H, Naim R (1993) Immunoglobulins or plasma exchange? Synchronization of plasma exchange and intravenous polyvalent immunoglobulins. A consecutive study of 11 patients. *Ann Med Interne (Paris)* 144 (8): 532–538

146 Euler HH, Krey U, Schroder O, Loffler H (1985) Membrane plasmapheresis technique in rats. Confirmation of antibody rebound. *J Immunol Methods* 84 (1–2): 313–319

147 Welcker M, Helmke K (1995) Therapy of autoimmune nephrotic glomerulopathies by combined immunoadsorption and IVIG therapy. *Immunität und Infektion* 23 (4): 140–141

T-cell directed treatment: anti-thymocyte globulin

Wilhelm H. Schmitt[1], Ernst C. Hagen[2] and Fokko J. van der Woude[1]

[1]Fifth Department of Medicine, University Hospital Mannheim of the University of Heidelberg, Theodor Kutzer Ufer 1–3, 68167 Mannheim, Germany; [2]Eemland Ziekenhuis, Locatie "Lichtenberg", Dept. of Internal Medicine, Utrechtsweg 160, 3818 ES Amersfoort, The Netherlands

Introduction: T cells and ANCA associated vasculitis

Untreated, Wegener's granulomatosis (WG) and microscopic polyangiitis (MPA), the most important ANCA-associated systemic vasculitides (AASV), commonly take a lethal course or result in severe permanent organ damage. Although the majority of cases does respond to daily oral cyclophosphamide and corticosteroids [1], the standard induction therapy fails to induce remission in about 5% to 10% of patients. Furthermore, relapses occur in 10% to 20% of patients within 12 months after successful induction of remission and indicate a poorer long-term prognosis. The usual therapeutic management of such cases is prolonged administration or re-administration of cyclophosphamide. In frequent relapsers this will often lead to high cumulative doses. The risk for severe side-effects of cyclophosphamide, e.g., malignancies, bone-marrow toxicity and hemorrhagic cystitis, increases dramatically in patients with a cumulative dose higher than 100 g [2]. There is a definite need to replace cyclophosphamide in these refractory cases. In other patients, standard treatment has to be avoided because severe side-effects already developed. Few patients have been reported to have responded to Cyclosporin A [3], intravenous immunoglobulins [4] or humanized antibodies against lymphocyte antigens (CAM-PATH) [5, 6]. However, the number of reported patients is low, and these drugs have never been studied in controlled trials.

There is increasing evidence for a pathogenetic role of T cells in AASV, especially in anti-proteinase 3 positive WG, recently summarised by Franssen et al. [7] and Harper and Savage [8]: In both WG and MPA, T cells have been demonstrated in active vasculitic lesions in renal, lung and nasal biopsies [9, 10], and there is evidence for a bias towards a TH1 cytokine profile [10]. Enhanced expression of chemokines and adhesion molecules involved in T-cell recruitment has been

Disease-modifying Therapy in Vasculitides, edited by Cees G. M. Kallenberg and
Jan W. Cohen Tervaert
© 2001 Birkhäuser Verlag Basel/Switzerland

demonstrated in active vasculitic lesions (for an overview see [8]). There is evidence from *in vitro* studies that T-helper cells and peripheral blood mononuclear cells from patients with WG proliferate on stimulation with proteinase 3 [11–13]. The antigen-specific T cells persist in the peripheral blood during periods of remission [12]. In contrast to anti-PR3 associated vasculitis, only one [13] of three studies [11–13] has reported T-cell proliferation in response to myeloperoxidase in anti-myeloperoxidase positive patients. It has been speculated whether such T cells participate in the pathogenesis of vasculitis at initiation and effector stages of the immune response, but formal proof is lacking. The presence of antigen-specific T cells at vasculitic tissue sites has not yet been demonstrated. However, elevated levels of T-cell activation markers such as soluble interleukin 2 receptor and soluble CD30 have been described in WG and Churg-Strauss syndrome and were shown to correlate with clinical disease activity. Levels remain elevated in remission, although conventional sero-markers of disease activity may have returned to the normal range [14–17]. Relapses in patients with WG are often associated with or preceded by rising levels of these markers [14, 17]. In active anti-MPO-ANCA positive patients, plasma levels of sCD30 were described to be lower than in the anti-PR3 positive subgroup [18]. Furthermore, T-cell activation implies involvement of MHC molecules: In most cases of T-cell dependent autoimmune diseases there are clear positive or negative associations with HLA class II antigens. In AASV, a protective effect of HLA DR6/HLA DR13 for both PR3- and MPO-ANCA positive cases is the only confirmed finding [19, 20]. Otherwise, the search for associations of HLA class II alleles with AASV has produced conflicting results.

Finally, also in non-ANCA-associated vasculitis such as giant cell arteritis, there is strong evidence for the involvement of T cells as demonstrated by studies of temporal arteries from giant cell arteritis patients that were implanted into SCID mice. Again, a TH1 cytokine pattern was demonstrated [21, 22].

In summary, there is enough evidence for a pathogenetic role of T cells in systemic vasculitis to justify anti T-cell directed experimental therapeutic designs in patients with refractory AASV or patients who cannot be treated with standard therapy due to severe side-effects.

Anti-thymocyte globulin (ATG)

Polyclonal anti-lymphocyte globulin and anti-thymocyte globulin (ATG) preparations have been available for more than 20 years and have been used successfully for reversing acute allograft rejections [23–25]. ATG is produced by injecting animals, usually horses or rabbits, with human T cells to prepare purified gamma globulin fractions of the resulting immune sera. The sources of antigens differ: thymic or thoracic duct cells or continuous T-cell lines (e.g. Jurkatt cells) are used as immunogens. *In vivo*, administration of ATG is followed by a profound lymphocytopenia of rapid onset [26]. Although lymphocyte counts recover within days to weeks after cessation of treatment, T cells that reappear are functionally impaired and their proliferative response remains reduced so that immunosuppression lasts on. Mechanisms of action of ATG include classic complement-mediated lysis of lymphocytes, clearance of lymphocytes due to reticuloendothelial uptake, masking of T-cell antigens, or expansion of negative regulatory cells [27]. However, ATG always represents a heterogeneous group of antibodies, only a minority of which are specific for T cells, and different preparations may vary considerably with respect to their immunosuppressive properties.

Published experience with ATG in vasculitis

Although there is a convincing rationale to use ATG in vasculitis, published experience is restricted to two case reports and one pilot study: The pilot study published by Hagen et al. in 1995 consisted of five patients with severe, refractory active Wegener's granulomatosis [28]. Previously, all patients had been treated with cyclophosphamide and steroids, two of them for more than 5 years. Three patients were unresponsive to standard therapy, and two had developed severe side-effects. Rabbit-anti-human ATG (Rijksinstituut voor Volksgezondheit en Millieuhygiene, Bilthoven, The Netherlands) was given for up to 10 days at an initial dose of 5 mg/kg body weight. The peripheral blood lymphocyte count was monitored daily to assess the effect of treatment and to adjust subsequent doses of ATG. Four of five patients showed a favorable response, with partial ($n = 3$) or complete ($n = 1$) remission of disease activity, during a follow-up period of 5 to 12 months. Interestingly, granulomatous lesions such as orbital pseudotumors and nasal/sinus granulomata (improvement at one of three sites of active disease) did not respond as good as vascular lesions (episcleritis and glomerulonephritis; improvement at five of five sites of active disease). Subsequent steroid doses could be reduced in all four responders, and all except two patients were free of other immunosuppressive agents. The cANCA became negative in three of four responders. A subsequent case report on one of these five patients showed that this particular patient finally remained free of active disease for 5.5 years, and was off any immunosuppressive treatment for about 3.5 years [29].

Another case report described a leucocytopenic patient suffering of severe pANCA associated microscopic polyangiitis (pulmonary renal syndrome, dialysis dependent), who was successfully treated with corticosteroid pulses and ATG (clinical remission, off dialysis) [30]. In addition to these cases, ATG has been successfully administered in patients with refractory SLE, systemic sclerosis, rheumatoid arthritis and autoimmune haemolytic anaemia. However, published experience in these disorders is restricted to two case reports [31, 32].

The SOLUTION protocol of the EUVAS group: ATG in refractory ANCA associated SV

In order to identify patients who are likely to respond to ATG-treatment, the European Vasculitis Study Group (EUVAS) launched an open, multicentre study (SOLUTION protocol) to investigate the efficacy and side-effects of ATG-treatment in patients with AASV, who cannot receive standard therapy. Two groups of patients qualify for this trial: (1) patients with progressive AASV unresponsive to or intolerant of standard treatment with cytotoxic agents and systemic corticosteroids. The primary endpoint is induction of remission. (2) patients with constant grumbling disease who tend to relapse after reduction or omission of cytotoxic agents and who experienced severe side-effects due to these drugs. Maintenance of remission after ATG and dose-reduction of other immunosuppressants are the primary end-points. Active disease as well as partial and complete remission are diagnosed according to predefined definitions.

Patients initially receive 2.5 mg/kg body weight of rabbit anti-human ATG (Thymoglobulin Merieux, Lyon, France). During a 10-day regimen, further doses are adjusted to lymphocyte counts. To prevent allergy, all patients receive 100 mg methylprednisolone before the first administration of ATG, and azathioprine (2 mg/kg) is given throughout the ATG-treatment. After the course of ATG, the further use of immunosuppressive drugs follows clinical demands and local practice.

The study is still going on, and further patients can be included. So far, 11 cases all suffering of severe, histologically proven Wegener's granulomatosis have been treated within or according to the protocol. Six were unresponsive to daily oral cyclophosphamide, and five were intolerant of this regime (hemorrhagic cystitis in three, leucopenia in one, hepatotoxicity in one). Before ATG administration, patients had received a mean of four (two to six) different therapeutic approaches including oral cyclophosphamide in all and multiple experimental therapies in four (mycophenolate mofetil in four, intravenous immunoglobulin in three, deoxyspergualin in two), without control of disease activity (3.5 ± 2 relapses during a disease duration of 73 ± 54 months). When ATG was given, all patients had active disease involving a mean of 2.5 (one to four) organ systems (Tab. 1). Patients received a mean of two (two to five) infusions of ATG with a total dose of 340 mg (190–500 mg). Nine out of 10 patients showed a favorable response to ATG with partial ($n = 9$) or complete ($n = 1$) remission of disease activity (Tab. 1). After ATG administration, remaining disease activity was restricted to one (zero to two) organ system. Although further immunosuppressive treatment was required in all, a dose reduction or a change to a less aggressive regime could be achieved in nine cases. Noteworthy is that in all six patients who were treated with cyclophosphamide directly before ATG administration this drug could be stopped thereafter. However, it should be stressed that the response to ATG in some patients occurred only after an interval of several weeks. This is in concordance with previous experience [28].

Table 1 - Patients treated with ATG within the SOLUTION protocol (EUVAS group)

Patient No.	Disease extent at ATG administration (ELK-classification)[1]	Disease extent after ATG administration (ELK-classification)[1]	Therapy[2] directly before ATG	Therapy[2] after ATG	Duration of remission (months)	Clinical relapse (ELK-classification)[1]
1	E, L, B	L unchanged	CYC,T/S,GC	MMF, GC	2	Ey
2	Ey, P	Ey better, P →	CYA, GC	MMF, GC	24	none
3	E, L, B	L improved	DSG, GC	MMF, GC	5	none
4	K	K improved	CYC, GC	MMF, GC	12	none
5	L, B	L improved	MMF, GC	MMF, GC	2.5	S, A
6	L	L improved	CYC, GC	T/S, GC	15	none
7	K, A, P	K improved	CYC	AZA, GC	29	K
8	L, K, B	died L	CYC, GC	–	–	–
9	E,L,K,B	E + L improved	CYC, GC	AZA, GC	12	none
10	L, K	L + K improved	IVIG	CYA, GC	14	L
11	K, A, P	none	MMF,GC	MMF, a-TNF, GC	6	none

[1]*ELK-classification to assess disease extent: E, ENT region; L, lungs; K, kidneys; P, polyneuropathy; A, arthritis, arthralgia, myalgia; B, constitutional symptoms; → = unchanged*
[2]*Therapies: CYC, cyclophosphamide; GC, glucocorticosteroids; IVIG, intravenous immunoglobulins; AZA, azathioprine; MMF, mycophenolate mofetil; DSG, deoxyspergualin; CYA, cyclosporin A; T/S, trimethoprim/sufamethoxazole; a-TNF, anti-TNFα directed therapy (eternacept)*
EUVAS, European Vasculitis Study Group

Currently, six patients are free of relapse for 10 (3–28) months. ANCA became negative in three, and titers were reduced in three further patients (no data on five cases). One patient died due to active WG 3 days after ATG administration (pulmonary hemorrhage). During a follow-up of 17 ± 11 months, four patients relapsed after 12 (2–29) months. Two of the four relapses occurred at sites not affected by active vasculitis/granuloma formation at the time of ATG administration. CD4 counts remained reduced (data available for six patients only). It could be argued that concomitant treatment with glucocorticosteroids added to the favorable response. However, it is known that moderate doses of corticosteroids alone (up to 20 mg in the cases of this study) are not capable to induce or maintain remission in WG. Therefore, treatment with ATG must have contributed to the significant improvement seen in these cases of refractory disease.

Table 2 - Adverse effects of ATG treatment

Adverse effects	Frequency	Reference
Fever, chills, headache during first infusion	> 90%	[27, 28]
Serum sickness	10–20%	[23, 24, 28]
Anaphylactoid reactions	associated with previous application of foreign globulin, exclude pre-sensitisation by intradermal testing	[27, 28]
Mild thrombocytopenia, granulocytopenia	common	[27]
Increased incidence of opportunistic infections, especially cytomegalovirus and herpes simplex	frequency increased with profound lymphocytopenia and aggressive immuno-suppressive therapy	[27, 28, 34]
Malignancies	increased incidence of lymphoma and Kaposi's sarcoma	[36]
Acute renal failure	rare	[37]

Side-effects of ATG treatment

Side-effects of ATG treatment are summarized in Table 2. As known from previous experience [28], all patients treated within the SOLUTION protocol experienced fever and chills associated with the first application of ATG. Further side-effects were restricted to a minority of cases: One patient suffered of serum sickness, clinically manifested with arthralgias, purpura and fever 13 days after the first ATG administration. The condition dramatically improved after two plasma exchanges without any further immunosuppressive therapy. The patient was positive for IgM rheumatoid factor, which is frequently present in active WG and may cross react with rabbit IgG [33]. Serum sickness was previously observed in two of five WG patients treated with ATG [28] and is known to occur in about 10% of renal transplant patients after ATG administration [24]. Further side-effects associated with unwanted antibodies to polyclonal antibody medications include thrombocytopenia and granulocytopenia. Because of the development of host antibodies to the non-human globulin, anaphylactoid reactions can occur [27]. Therefore, the use of rabbit ATG is contraindicated in patients who previously received rabbit immunoglobulins. The application of horse ATG may be an alternative in these cases. A pre-sensitization of the patient against rabbit/horse globulin must be excluded by intradermal testing with ATG in advance of systemic ATG administration to avoid severe anaphylactoid reactions.

Although no life-threatening infections were seen in AASV patients treated with ATG, opportunistic infections associated with ATG therapy have been of major concern especially in transplant recipients. Cytomegalovirus (CMV) infection occurred in only one of the patients treated within the SOLUTION protocol but is frequently associated with ATG treatment after transplantation of allografts. Furthermore, it is known that the course of CMV disease is aggravated after ATG administration, and failure of ganciclovir prophylaxis to eradicate CMV has recently been associated with ATG in renal transplant recipients [34]. One of the patients treated within the SOLUTION protocol developed an abscess of a labium majus (*Staphylococcus aureus*) 3 weeks after ATG administration that required surgical drainage. A causal relationship to ATG treatment seems likely, and abscess formation has been described previously in association with this form of therapy [35]. Furthermore, follow-up studies after kidney transplantation demonstrate that ATG treatment increases the risk for malignant disorders such as lymphoma and Kaposi's sarcoma [36]. Recently, a single high dose regimen of ATG (9 mg/kg) has been successfully employed in renal transplantation [37]. However, it is unknown whether this regime is applicable in AASV, and it remains to be confirmed whether side-effects can thus be reduced.

Conclusion

Although experience with ATG in patients with refractory AASV is still limited, summarized data obtained from previous studies and from the larger group of patients treated within the SOLUTION protocol indicate that ATG may be a treatment option for patients who do not respond to or tolerate standard therapy. Of a total of 17 patients treated so far, 15 responded, and further immunosuppressive therapy could be reduced in 13 (Tab. 3). Some of these patients experienced long lasting periods of remission although a minority later relapsed. With few exceptions, ATG treatment was well tolerated, and life-threatening side-effects did not occur. The response to ATG further supports the concept that T cells play a pathogenetic role in AASV. This is in line with other case reports demonstrating sustained improvement of various vasculitides such as microscopic polyangiitis and Behçet's disease after anti-T-cell directed treatment with anti-CDw52 anti-CD4 monoclonal antibodies [5, 6]. In contrast to these antibodies, which could only be used by a few centers with the necessary expertise to manage the side-effects, renal physicians are well acquainted with the usage of ATG for prophylaxis or treatment of renal-transplant rejections. ATG could therefore become a wider-spread therapeutic approach for AASV patients who cannot be treated by conventional means, and it seems justified to further study the effects of ATG on this disorder. As the SOLUTION pro-

Table 3 - Summarised experience with ATG in refractory AASV

Reference	Number of cases (n)	Diagnosis	Remission: partial (n)	complete (n)	Dose reduction of immunosuppressants (n)
[28]	5	all WG	4	none	4
[29], follow up of [28]	1	WG	–	1	yes
[30]	1	MPA	1	–	?
EUVAS group (SOLUTION)	11	all WG	9	1	9

WG, Wegener's granulomatosis; MPA, microscopic polyangiitis; EUVAS, European Vasculitis Study Group

tocol of the European Vasculitis Study Group is still recruiting patients, patients in whom ATG is considered should receive this drug in a standardized controlled fashion in order to define the place of ATG treatment in patients with refractory AASV.

References

1   Fauci AS, Haynes BF, Katz P, Wolff SM (1983) Wegener's granulomatosis: prospective clinical and therapeutic experience with 85 patients for 21 years. *Ann Intern Med* 98: 76–85

2   Hoffman GS, Kerr GS, Leavitt RY, Hallahan CW, Labovicz R, Travis WD, Rottem M Fauci AS (1992) Wegener's granulomatosis: an analysis of 158 patients *Ann Intern Med* 116: 488

3   Borleffs JCC, Derksen RHWM, Hene RJ (1987) Treatment of Wegener's granulomatosis with cyclosporin. *Ann Rheum Dis* 46: 175

4   Jayne DRW, Esnault VLM, Lockwood CM (1993) ANCA idiotype antibodies and the treatment of systemic vasculitis with intravenous immunglobulin. *J Autoimmun* 6: 207–219

5   Lockwood CM, Thiru S, Isaacs J, Hale G, Waldman H (1993) Long-term remission of intractable systemic vasculitis with monoclonal antibody therapy. *Lancet* 341: 1620

6   Mathieson PW, Cobbold SP, Hale G, Clark MR, Oliveira DBG, Lockwood CM, Waldman H (1990) Monoclonal antibody therapy in systemic vasculitis. *N Engl J Med* 323: 250

7   Franssen CFM, Stegeman CA, Kallenberg CGM, Gans ROB, De Jong PE, Hoorntje SJ,

Cohen Tervaert JW (2000) Antiproteinase 3- and antimyeloperoxidase associated vasculitis. *Kidney Int* 57: 2195–2206

8   Harper L, Savage COS (2000) Pathogenesis of ANCA-associated vasculitis. *J Pathol* 190: 349–359

9   Bolton WK, Innes D, Sturgill BC, Kaiser DL (1987) T cells and macrophages in rapidly progressive glomerulonephritis: Clinicopathological correlates. *Kidney Int* 32: 869–876

10   Csernok E, Trabandt A, Müller A, Wang GC, Moosig F, Pailsen J, Schnabel A, Gross WL (1999) Cytokine profiles in Wegener's granulomatosis: predominace of type 1 (Th1) in the granulomatous inflammation. *Arthritis Rheum* 42: 742–750

11   Brouwer E, Stegeman C, Muitema M, Limburg PC, Kallenberg CGM (1994) T-cell reactivity to proteinase 3 and myeloperoxidase in patients with Wegener's granulomatosis. *Clin Exp Immunol* 98: 448–453

12   King WJ, Brooks CJ, Holder R, Hughes P, Adu D, Savage COS (1998) T lymphocyte responses to anti-neutrophil cytoplasmic antibody (ANCA) antigens are present in patients with ANCA associated systemic vasculitis and persist during disease remission. *Clin Exp Immunol* 112: 539–546

13   Griffith ME, Coulhart A, Pusey CD (1996) T-cell responses to myeloperoxidase (MPO) and proteinase 3 (PR3) in patients with systemic vasculitis. *Clin Exp Immunol* 103: 253–258

14   Schmitt WH, Heesen C, Csernok E, Rautmann A, Gross WL (1992) Elevated serum levels of soluble interleukin-2 receptor in patients with Wegener's granulomatosis. *Arthritis Rheum* 35: 1088–1096

15   Schmitt WH, Csernok E, Kobayashi S, Klinkenborg A, Reinhold-Keller E, Gross WL (1998) Churg-Strauss syndrome: serum markers of lymphocyte activation and endothelial damage. *Arthritis Rheum* 41: 445–452

16   Wang G, Csernok E, Gross WL (1997) High plasma levels of the soluble form of CD30 activation molecule reflect disease activity in patients with Wegener's granulomatosis. *Am J Med* 102: 517–523

17   Stegeman CA, Cohen Tervaert JW, Huittema MG, Kallenberg CGM (1993) Serum markers of T-cell activation in relapses of Wegener's granulomatosis. *Clin Exp Immunol* 91: 415–420

18   Franssen CFM, Oost-Kort WW, Stegeman CA, Kallenberg CGM, Cohen Tervaert JW (1988) Markers of T-cell and monocyte activation in antiproteinase 3 and antimyeloperoxidase associated crescentic glomerulonephritis, in anti-proteinase 3 and anti-myeloperoxidase associated dystemic vasculitis: differences in clinical presentation and pathophysiology. Thesis, CFM Franssen, Groningen, 103–115

19   Hagen EC, Stegeman CA, D'Amaro J, Schreuder GMT, van Es LA, Cohen Tervaert JW, Kallenberg CGM, van der Woude FJ (1995) Decreased frequency of HLA DR13DR6 in Wegener's granulomatosis. *Kid Int* 48: 801–805

20   Gencik M, Borgmann S, Zahn R, Albert E, Sitter T, Epplein JT, Fricke H (1999) Immunogenic risk factors for anti-neutrophil cytoplasmic antibody (ANCA)-associated systemic vasculitis. *Clin Exp Immunol* 117: 412–417

21 Brack A, Geisler A, Martinez-Taboada V, Younge B, Goronzy J, Weyand C (1997) Giant cell vasculitis is a T-cell dependent disease. *Mol Med* 3: 530–543

22 Weyand CM, Hicok KC, Hunder GG, Goronzy JJ (1994) Tissue cytokine patterns in patients with polymyalgia rheumatica and giant cell arteritis. *Ann Inter Med* 121: 726–728

23 Hoitsma AJ, Reekers P, Kreftenberg JG, van Lier HJJ, Capel PJA, Koene RAP (1982) Treatment of acute rejection of cadaveric renal allografts with rabbit anticymocyte globulin. *Transplantation* 33: 12

24 Hoitsma AJ, van Lier HJJ, Reekers P, Koene RAP (1985) Improved patients and graft survival after treatment of acute rejections of cadaveric renal allografts with rabbit anticymocyte globulin. *Transplantation* 39: 274

25 Lamich R, Bakkester M, Marti V, Brossa V, Aymat R, Carrio I, Berna L, Camprecios M, Puig M, Estorch M et al (1998) Efficacy of augmented immunosuppressive therapy for early vasculopathy in heart transplantation. *J Am Coll Cardiol* 32: 413–419

26 Mestre M, Bas J, Alsina J, Grinyo JM, Buendia E (1999) Depleting effects of antithymocyte globulin on T-lymphocyte subsets in kidney transplantation. *Transplant Proc* 31: 2254–2255

27 Burdick JF (1986) The biology of immunosuppression mediated by anti-lymphocyte antibodies. In: GM William, JF Burdick, K Solez K (eds): *Kidney transplant rejection: diagnosis and treatment*. Marcel Dekker, New York, 307–312

28 Hagen EC, De Keizer RJW, Andrassy K, van Boven WPL, Bruijn JA, van ES LA, van der Woude FJ (1995) Compassionate treatment of Wegener's granulomatosis with rabbit anti-thymocyte globulin. *Clin Nephrol* 43: 351–359

29 Kool J, de Keizer RJW, Siegert CEH (1999) Antithymocyte globulin treatment of orbital Wegener granulomatosis: a follow-up study. *Am J Opthalmol* 127: 738–739

30 Lukas R, Keller F (1998) Anti-thymocyte globulin therapy in a patient with pANCA vasculitis and crescentic glomerulonephritis (letter). *Nephron* 78: 231

31 Tarkowski A, Anderson-Gare B, Aurell M (1993) Use of anti-thymocyte globulin in the management of refractory systemic autoimmune diseases. *Scand J Rheumatol* 22: 261–266

32 Tarkowski A, Lindgren I (1994) Beneficial effects of antithymocyte globulin in severe cases of progressive systemic sclerosis. *Transplant Proceed* 26: 3197–3199

33 van der Woude FJ, Daha MR, van den Wall Bake WA, van ES LA (1990) Antibodies directed against the cytoplasm of neutrophils and monocytes. *Adv Nephrol Necker Hosp* 19: 211–214

34 Isenberg AL, Shen GK, Singh TP, Hahn A, Conti DJ (2000) Failure of ganciclovir prophylaxis to completely eradicate CMV disease in renal transplant recipients treated with intense anti-rejection immunotherapy. *Clin Transplant* 14: 193–198

35 Morishita Y, Matsukawa Y, Kura Y, Takei M, Tomita Y, Nishinarita S, Horie T (1997) antithymocyte globulin for a patient with systemic lupus erythematosus complicated by severe pancytopenia. *J Int Med Res* 25: 219–223

36 Farge D, Lebbe C, Marjanovic Z, Tuppin P, Mouquet C, Peraldi NN, Lang P, Hiesse C,

Antoine C, Legendre C, Bedrossian J et al (1999) Human herpes virus-8 and other risk factors for Kaposi's sarcoma in kidney transplant recipients. Group Cooperatif de Transplantation d'Ile de France (GCIF). *Transplantation* 67: 1236–1242

37   Samsel R, Chmura R, Wlodarczyk Z, Wyzgal J, Cieciura T, Lagiewska B, Piszczinski J, Korczak G, Lasowski T, Paczek L et al (1999) Perioperative single high dose ATG-Fresenius S administration as induction immunosuppressive therapy in cadaveric renal transplantation–preliminary results. *Ann Transplant* 4: 37–39

38   Levine JM, Lien YH (1999) Antithymocyte globulin-induced acute renal failure (letter). *Am J Kidney Dis* 34: 1155

New immunosuppressants: mycophenolate mofetil and 15-deoxyspergualin

Coen A. Stegeman[1] and Rainer Birck[2]

[1]Department of Internal Medicine, Division of Nephrology, University Hospital Groningen, Hanzeplein 1, 9713 GZ Groningen, The Netherlands; [2]V. Medizinische Klinik, Nephrologie/Endokrinologie, Universitätsklinikum Mannheim, Theodor-Kutzer-Ufer 1–3, 68167 Mannheim, Germany

Introduction

Primary or idiopathic vasculitic syndromes are a group of inflammatory disorders of presumed autoimmune origin characterized by inflammation of blood vessels leading to vessel wall necrosis and (partial) obliteration or thrombosis of the vascular lumen. Clinical signs and symptoms are caused by disruption of adequate macro- and microcirculatory blood flow of organs or tissues by the vascular inflammatory proces. The classification of these idiopathic systemic vasculitic syndromes is based on the size and localization of the vessels predominantly involved and certain characteristics of the histopathology of the inflammatory process [1]. Several different classification schemes have been proposed, the latest modification being the scheme set up by a Consensus Conference in Chapel Hill in 1992 (Tab. 1) [2]. The factors involved in the pathogenesis of primary vasculitides are as yet unidentified. The possible autoimmune origin of these diseases is supported by the strong association of the presence of autoantibodies directed against neutrophil cytoplasmic antigens, so-called anti-neutrophil cytoplasmic antibodies (ANCA), in some of the primary small vessel vasculitides [2, 3].

Standard treatment of primary vasculitis

In addition to supportive therapy, treatment of primary vasculitic syndromes is based on immunosuppressive therapy with corticosteroids with or without alkylating or anti-metabolite compounds such as cyclophosphamide, chlorambucil, azathioprine or methotrexate. Although individual exceptions occur, some of the primary vasculitic syndromes generally respond adequately to (high dose) corticosteroids only and remission can be maintained with low doses of corticosteroids. In giant cell arteriitis, Takayashu's arteriitis and cases of Henoch-Schönlein purpura that are not self-limiting, additional therapy is usually not needed [4, 5]. In classic ANCA and hepatitis B negative polyarteritis nodosa addition of cyclophosphamide

Table 1 - Classification of systemic idiopathic vasculitides according to the Chapel Hill Consensus Conference [2]

I. Large vessel vasculitis
   1. Takayasu's arteritis
   2. Giant cell arteritis/temporal arteritis

II. Medium-sized vessel vasculitis
   1. (Classic) polyarteritis nodosa
   2. Kawasaki disease

III. Small vessel vasculitis
   1. Wegener's granulomatosis[1]
   2. Churg-Strauss syndrome[1]
   3. Microscopic polyangiitis[1]
   4. Henoch-Schönlein purpura
   5. Essential cryoglobulinemic vasculitis
   6. Cutaneous leukocytoclastic vasculitis

[1]*strongly associated with anti-neutrophil cytoplasmic autoantibodies*

does not improve survival, but does improve disease control [6, 7]. In addition, Kawasaki's disease responds to pooled intravenous gammaglobulin and acetylsalicylic acid [8, 9]. However, especially the ANCA related small vessel vasculitic syndromes do not respond to corticosteroids alone and standard therapy in these diseases includes the use of substantial doses of the alkylating agent cyclophosphamide for induction and maintenance of disease remission [10–13]. Given the high tendency for relapse in ANCA associated vasculitis with frequencies up to 50% or more within 5 years after diagnosis, cycloposphamide related short- and long-term toxicity is a substantial problem [13, 14]. Serious long-term sequelae of cyclophosphamide toxicity such as infertility and gonadal failure, bladder cancer, bone marrow failure, and the development of haematological or other malignancies develop after months or years of follow-up and are related to the cumulative dose of cyclophosphamide [13, 15–20]. Therefore, strategies to reduce this cumulative dose are being investigated.

Strategies to reduce treatment toxicity in ANCA related vasculitis

The actual and cumulative cyclophosphamide dose and related toxicity can be reduced by using intravenous pulse therapy. A meta-analysis of three published randomised clinical trials in active ANCA-related vasculitis shows that pulse as compared to continuous oral therapy is associated with an increased frequency of failure to induce remission and with a higher relapse rate, but with less infectious complications and leucopenia [21–24]. In less extensive cases of Wegener's granulomatosis without severe pulmonary or renal involvement remission induction with methotrexate and corticosteroids has been achieved [25–27]. In patients with Wegener's granulomatosis with disease activity limited to the upper or lower airways without signs of systemic vasculitis, some will respond to monotherapy with trimethoprim-sulfamethoxazole [28].

Another approach to reduce the amount of cyclophosphamide needed in patients with ANCA-related vasculitis is to limit its use to the induction phase. The early treatment schemes used daily oral cyclophosphamide in dosages of 1.5 to 2.0 mg/kg for 1 to 2 years [10, 11]. A recent prospective, randomized European study involving 155 newly diagnosed patients with Wegener's granulomatosis and microscopic polyangiitis showed that switching cyclophosphamide to azathioprine 3 to 6 months after remission induction is safe and does not lead to more relapses during follow-up for 2 years [29]. Whether this comparable efficacy is sustained during longer follow-up, or whether prolonged therapy with azathioprine is able to reduce the number of relapses is unclear. Others have described beneficial effects of maintenace therapy with methotrexate, cyclosporine A, or the addition of trimethoprim-sulfamethoxazole to reduce the frequency of relapses [30–32].

Potential new immunosuppressive drugs for treatment of active ANCA-related vasculitis

Currently, many patients with active ANCA-related vasculitis cannot be treated without cyclophosphamide despite its known toxicity. As a consequence of improved diagnosis and treatment of necrotizing small vessel vasculitis in the 1970s and 1980s, more patients in whom renewed treatment with cyclophosphamide is impossible due to cumulative toxicity survive to experience new episodes of active vasculitis. Physicians following these patients face the daunting task to treat these patients once disease activity relapses. Successful use of the alkylating agents chlorambucil or etoposide has been described in case reports [17, 33]. Since these latter drugs have toxicity profiles partly overlapping that of cyclophosphamide their potential is limited. Therefore, other immunosuppressive drugs with different toxicity profiles are needed. The newly (re-)discovered drugs 15-deoxyspergualin and mycophenolic acid may be candidates in this respect and the profiles of these drugs and data on its use in primary vasculitis will be discussed here in detail.

15-deoxyspergualin

Drug characteristics

15-Deoxyspergualin (DSG; 1-amino-19-guanidino-11hydroxy-4,9,12-triazanona-decane-10,1 3-dione; generic name gusperimus, Fig. 1) is a synthetic analogue of spergualin, a natural product of the soil bacterium Bacillus laterosporus. Spergualin, a peptidomimetic compound containing the polyamine spermidine within its structure was discovered in 1981 by Umezawa et al. in a culture filtrate while screening for natural products that inhibit the transformation of chicken embry fibroblasts through Rous sarcoma virus [34, 35]. The first preclinical studies with DSG focused on its antitumor properties in a variety of animal tumor models [36, 37] leading finally to phase I clinical trials at the National Cancer Institute in the late 1980s. DSG arrested the growth of leucemic cells, but no antitumor effects were observed in late stage solid tumours. In these phase I studies it was found that DSG is well tolerated at doses up to 2000 mg/m^2/day [37].

Subsequently, strong immunosuppressive properties of DSG were discovered in several animal models. *In vivo* studies demonstrated prolongation of transplant allograft survival [38–40], induction of transplant tolerance [41], reversal of ongoing allograft rejection [42], and inhibition of autoimmune disease development including models of systemic lupus erythematodes and anti-GBM-nephritis [43], blocking of antibody responses [44–46] as well as suppression of delayed-type hypersensitivity [47].

Between 1988 to 1994, 436 patients experiencing acute renal allograft rejection were treated with DSG in Japan. In 76% of the cases rejection was successfully reversed, and based on these data registration was granted 1994 in Japan. Since then 2250 cases of acute rejection have been treated with DSG in Japan showing 73% efficacy, the major side-effect being transient leucopenia [48].

Mechanism of action: *in vitro* studies

DSG exerts its immunosuppressive effects by a mode of action not yet completely understood. The interaction with the immune system is not comparable with other immunosuppressants such as the immunophilins cyclosporine A or tacrolimus, or nucleotide synthesis inhibitors like azathioprine, mycophenolate mofetil or leflunamide.

Despite rather poor inhibition of T-cell proliferation *in vitro* in response to mitogens or alloantigens, DSG can inhibit mixed lymphocyte reactions even when added up to 48 h after the initiation [49]. DSG also blocks the development of cytotoxic T lymphocytes, but does not affect the effector phase of CTL-assays [49]. Interest-

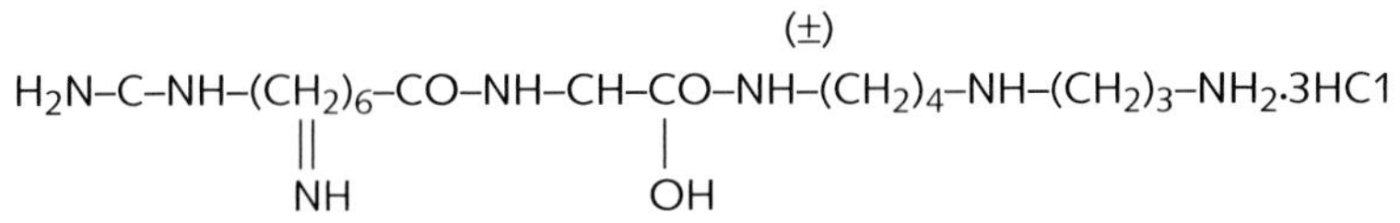

(±)

$H_2N–C–NH–(CH_2)_6–CO–NH–CH–CO–NH–(CH_2)_4–NH–(CH_2)_3–NH_2.3HC1$

$\quad\quad\; \| \quad\quad\quad\quad\quad\quad\quad\quad |$

$\quad\quad NH \quad\quad\quad\quad\quad\quad\quad OH$

Molecular formula: $C_{17}H_{37}N_7O_3.3HCl$

Molecular weight: 496.91

Figure 1
Chemical structure of 15-deoxyspergualin

ingly, Nemoto et al. recently reported that DSG was found to induce apoptotic cell death [50].

A consistent finding is the potent inhibition of both primary and secondary humoral immune responses by DSG. Immunoglobulin synthesis by B cells triggered by T-cell dependent and T-cell-independent antigens is inhibited [45, 46]. However, DSG does not inhibit B cell proliferation [51] or the secretion of immunoglobulins in B cell myelomas or hybridomas [52]. The effect on antibody production may be explained by the inhibition of B-cell differentiation and κ light chain expression at a transcriptional level by blocking nuclear translocation of the transcription factor NF-κB by DSG [53]. In addition, in mice DSG leads to an arrest of T-lymphocyte maturation in the thymus during $CD4^-CD8^-$ to $CD4^+CD8^+$ transition as well as to an arrest in B lymphocytes during pre-B-cell differentiation in the bone marrow when the prereceptor complex containing the immunoglobulin heavy chain is expressed, while mature T or B cells appeared unaffected [54]. From these data it appears that DSG rather affects differentiation than proliferation of lymphocytes.

In monocyte/macrophage/antigen presenting cells DSG has been shown to decrease the generation of reactive oxygen species and hydrolytic enzymes [55]. Immunhistological staining shows that expression of MHC class I and II antigens [56] as well as proliferation and antigen processing/presentation are qualitatively affected [57, 58].

A major breakthrough was the recent discovery that DSG binds to an intracellular chaperone, the constitutively expressed cytoplasmic member of the heat shock protein family Hsc70 [59]. The binding constants for Hsc70 have been shown to be within the range of pharmacologic levels of DSG *in vivo*. Moreover, the immunosuppressive activity of DSG and related analogues correlates with their binding affinities for Hsc70 *in vitro* [60]. Since heat shock proteins act as molecular chaperones for intracellular polypeptides [61] and may be necessary for antigen processing as well as for translocation of nuclear transcription factors [62], these findings provide a clue for the understanding of the action of DSG at the molecular level.

Pharmacokinetics and toxicology

The pharmacokinetics of DSG have been studied in various preclinical animal experiments [63, 64] as well as in patients with advanced cancer [37], renal transplants [65], multiple sclerosis and rheumatoid arthritis [66, 67]. No pharmacokinetic differences could be detected between Caucasians and Japanese [68]. DSG exhibits a bi-exponential decay in plasma with an initial half-life of 5–60 min and a terminal elimination half-life of approximately 2 h (range 0.75–14 h) and is metabolized to several metabolites which are neither immunosuppressive nor toxic [69, 70]. Only 10% of the administered drug is eliminated unchanged in the urine [69]. The unmetabolized drug fraction does not accumulate in the presence of impaired renal function [71, 72], or during prolonged administration four times weekly of 0.25 mg/kg s.c. for 16 weeks [73]. Since the oral availability of DSG is only 3–6% [71], the drug has to be given either i.v. or s.c. The average bioavailability after s.c. administration is consistently greater than 90% [74].

Preclinincal toxicology studies used for registration in Japan (1994), reveal no mutagenicity [75–83], teratogenicity [84–88] or cancerogenicity [89]. However, the drug is myelostatic to bone marrow stem cells leading to a transient, non-cumulative reversible bone marrow suppression in preclinical and clinical studies [63, 64].

Phase I studies in patients with advanced cancer showed no real antitumor properties, but important toxicological data were obtained. DSG was given as monotherapy in 190 patients in doses up to 2–75 mg/kg/day delivered by a 3- or 24-h infusion for 5 days. The main adverse effects were reversible hypotension and transient perioral numbness at the higher dose ranges. Mild myelosuppression was also observed. Importantly, DSG showed no diabetogenic, hepatoxic or nephrotoxic properties in this setting [37, 64]. In renal transplant patients with acute rejection, who receive DSG in doses of 3 to 5 mg/kg i.v. for 5 to 14 days, the drug is tolerated well. The most notable side-effect has been reversible leucopenia with a nadir occuring between 14 and 21 days after initiating DSG therapy. In an adverse side-effect report on 385 cases of acute renal allograft treated with DSG in 1998 to the Japanese health authorities leucopenia was reported in 35%, thrombocytopenia in 35%, anaemia in 14% [48]. A total of 38 infections without severe septicemia were observed in these patients [48]. In a randomized double-blind controlled study in multiple sclerosis in Germany and Switzerland, 236 patients were given DSG in doses of 2 mg/kg or 6 mg/kg i.v. in five 4-day courses at 4-week intervals. Despite a lack of efficacy, during the follow-up of 2 years the number and severity of adverse effects did not significantly differ from the placebo treated groups. During the treatment phases, a mild and transient myelosuppression with anemia and leucopenia was noted [90].

Clinical experience with DSG

Relevant experience in humans has been obtained in transplantation. DSG has shown an efficacy rate of 77% to 82% in the reversal of acute renal transplant rejection. In combination with methylprednisolone even an 94% efficacy rate was reported [91]. In steroid-resistant renal transplant rejection DSG was as effective as the monoclonal antibody OKT3 [92]. DSG was licensed in Japan in 1994 for treatment of acute renal allograft rejection. Since 1994 an estimated 2250 cases have been treated. In addition, DSG has been reported to be useful as part of induction therapy regimens in sensitized patients [93] and in ABO-incompatible combinations [94]. Anecdotal reports exist describing the succesful use of DSG in liver transplantation [95]. Furthermore, DSG succesfully prevented the production of antibodies (HAMAS) during administration of the mouse anti-colon-cancer antibody L6 during treatment raising the therapeutic response from 30% to greater than 90% [96].

Clinical data in ANCA-associated vasculitis

Since DSG is a potent immunosuppressant with a favorable side-effect profile, we decided to use it in patients with ANCA-associated vasculitis who do not tolerate or respond to standard treatment. Initially, in a pilot study two patients were treated, and after preliminary promising results [97], an ongoing open label multi center trial was initiated. Although several patients have been included in this study the follow-up is as yet too short to draw any conclusions. Therefore data from the first two patients treated in Mannheim will be discussed. Both patients suffered from biopsy proven Wegener's granulomatosis and were c-ANCA/anti-proteinase 3 positive.

The first patient, a 32-year-old male, was diagnosed with Wegener's granulomatosis in 1994. Initial presentation included pansinusitis, otitis media, arthralgias and myalgias. Unfortunately, 4 weeks after initiating therapy with cyclophosphamide and steroids, severe toxic hepatitis developed rendering further treatment with cyclophosphamide impossible. He was switched to azathioprine and despite short periods of improvement in between, the disease progressed relentlessly predominantly in the ENT region despite several immunosuppressive regimens including anti-thymocyte globulins. In May 1998, the patient showed progressive disease activity with new subglottic granulomata, hoarseness and constitutional symptoms under maintenance treatment with methotrexate and steroids. After obtaining informed consent, the patient was switched to DSG.

The second patient, a 48-year-old female, suffered from WG since 1995. She initially presented with otitis media, sinusitis, mononeuritis multiplex and necrotizing glomerulonephritis. She was treated with cyclophosphamide and steroids, but attempts to taper the cyclophosphamide dose resulted in frequent flare-ups of disease activity. Finally she was switched to mycophenolate mofetil, but in November 1998 she developed a new peroneal palsy and parethesias as well as progressive constitutional symptoms. Since she refused further treatment with cyclophosphamide we switched her to DSG after obtaining informed consent.

DSG (0.5 mg/kg/d) was given in both patients until a leucocyte nadir of 3.0×10^9/l was reached, adopting a therapeutical regime that had been used for treatment of various forms of proliferative glomerulonephritis by Hotta et al. [98]. Subsequently, DSG treatment was discontinued for 2 weeks to let leucocytes recover and the cycle was repeated. After the first week of i.v. DSG administration in hospital, treatment was continued s.c. in the same dosage to facilitate therapy in an outpatient setting. DSG treatment induced complete remission in both patients after three, respectively two treatment-cycles and was well tolerated. The patients remained in remission under maintenance therapy with DSG during the follow-up of 16 respectively 10 months so far. Besides reversible leucopenia no adverse effects were observed. Leucopenia occurred between day 14 and 20 of DSG treatment and followed in each patient a regular, almost predictable pattern during the cycles.

We conclude that DSG is able to induce and maintain complete remission in patients with active WG. Treatment was well tolerated and the expected main side-effect, leucopenia, was transient and foreseeable. No signs of cumulative toxicity after repeated cycles were seen as the pattern and duration of leucocyte depression did not change over time in the patients. Further studies are warranted to investigate DSG as secondary or even primary induction agent in patients with WG.

Mycophenolate mofetil

Drug characteristics

Mycophenolate mofetil is an organic synthetic derivate of the natural fermentation product of several *Penicillium* species' mycophenolic acid [99–101]. Mycophenolic acid is a potent, noncompetitive, reversible inhibitor of the enzyme inosine monophosphate dehydrogenase (IMPDH). In normal mammalian cells guanine and adenine nucleotides are produced from smaller precursors (*de novo* pathway), or by recycling of purine bases (salvage pathway) [102]. In the *de novo* pathway ribose 5-phosphate is converted in several steps involving 5-phosphoribosyl-1-pyrophosphate to inosine monophosphate (IMP). IMP is then converted to xanthine monophosphate by the enzyme IMPDH. The enzyme IMPDH exists in two isoforms, encoded by different genes. In contrast to many other cells, lymphocytes depend primarily on the *de novo* pathway for purine synthesis. Lymphocytes depleted of guanosine nucleotides become fixed in the S phase of the cell cycle and cannot proliferate [103]. In resting T and B lymphocytes the type I isoform of IMPDH is expressed, while activated proliferating T and B lymphocytes predominantly express the type II isoform. As mycophenolic acid has a five-fold higher binding affinity for IMPDH type II over type I, the result of the IMPDH inhibition is a rather selective inhibition of T and B lymphocyte proliferation with minimal effects on other systems [103–105]. Given these properties mycophenolic acid is an immunosuppressive drug with potentially a very favorable therapeutic window.

Pharmacokinetics and toxicity

Mycophenolate mofetil is an ester prodrug of the active compound mycophenolic acid necessary to increase bio-availability [100] (Fig. 2). After oral administration mycophenolate mofetil is rapidly and essentially completely absorbed [106, 107]. Once absorbed mycophenolate mofetil is rapidly hydrolized to mycophenolic acid [106] (Fig. 2). Following oral administration mycophenolate mofetil plasma levels are consequently below the limit of detection, while following intravenous administration the half-life time of mycophenolate mofetil is a few minutes [106, 107]. Oral bioavailability is > 90% and plasma peak levels of mycophenolic acid are reached within 1 h after administration [107]. Bioavailability is decreased with use of magnesium and aluminium hydroxide antacids and with cholysteramine. In plasma mycophenolic acid binds strongly to albumin (protein binding ~ 97%) and therefore the potential for drug interactions exists [108]. Mycophenolic acid is conjugated to glucuronide and is thereby inactivated. Mycophenolic acid glucuronide is eliminated in the urine, but is also partly excreted in the bile with subsequent enterohepatic recirculation following deconjugation in the intestinal tract resulting in a small rise in plasma levels of mycophenolic acid 8 to 12 h after administration [106, 109]. Around 70% of the dose of mycophenolate mofetil is recovered in the urine as mycophenolic acid glucuronide, while < 1% of the administered dose is recovered in the urine as mycophenolic acid. The terminal elimination half-life from plasma of mycophenolic acid is 17 h [107]. Although plasma levels of mycophenolic acid are not substantially influenced by renal failure, patients with compromised renal function have elevated levels of mycophenolic acid glucuronide. High plasma levels of mycophenolic acid glucuronide may increase the free fraction of mycophenolic acid by competing for the binding to plasma proteins, and thereby increase toxicity [110, 111].

Long-term use of mycophenolic acid is limited to 85 patients with psoriasis treated for up to 13 years [112]. Gastrointestinal side-effects including nausea, diarrhea, and cramping occurred in up to 75% of patients receiving 3 g mycophenolic acid

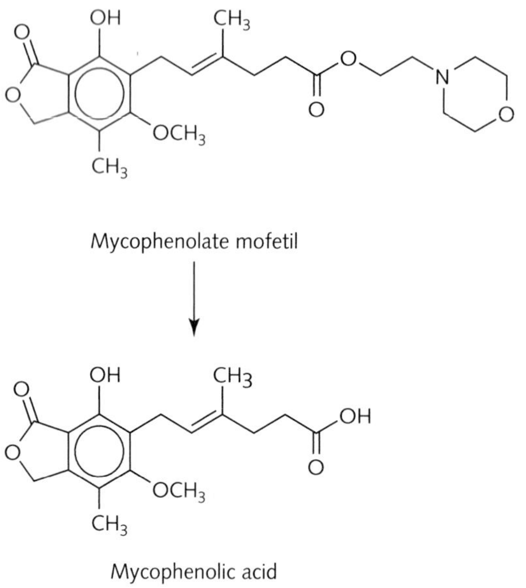

Figure 2
Chemical structure of mycophenolate mofetil and mycophenolic acid.

per day. With prolonged therapy the frequency of these side-effects dropped to 20%. Adverse effects observed in studies in renal transplant recipients involved the gastrointestinal tract and leukopenia and anaemia [113–116] Thrombocytopenia is very rare [116]. In a pooled analysis of the results of three randomized, double-blind clinical studies in renal transplant recipients adverse effects led to discontinuation of the study drug within the first year in 5.2%, 8.7%, and 14.7% in the placebo/ azathioprine (n = 492), mycophenolate mofetil 2 g/day (n = 501), and mycophenolate mofetil 3 g/day group (n = 490), respectively [116]. The frequency of opportunistic infections during the first year was slightly increased in the mycophenolate mofetil groups compared to placebo [113, 114], as was the case for tissue-invasive cytomegalovirus disease in patients treated with 3 g/day mycophenolate mofetil [109, 116, 117]. Although the studies do not have adequate power with respect to numbers and duration of follow-up to draw definite conclusions, at 3 years of follow-up the frequencies of lymphoproliferative disorders or other malignancies were not increased with mycophenolate mofetil therapy as compared to azathioprine [117].

Clinical experience with mycophenolate mofetil

Although mycophenolic acid is not a new drug, large scale clinical experience first dates from the second half of the 1990s. Randomized clinical trials have proven the efficacy of adding mycophenolate mofetil to standard therapy with cyclosporine A and corticosteroids in reducing the frequency and severity of acute rejection in renal transplantation with grafts both from cadaveric or living donors [113–118]. In this respect mycophenolate mofetil is more effective than azathioprine at the costs of only marginally increased incidences of treatment related gastrointestinal side-effects and opportunistic infections [114–117]. Moreover, in renal transplantation mycophenolate mofetil 2 g/day has been proven to have the superior treatment profile, as 3 g/day does not lead to further significant reductions in acute renal allograft rejection while increasing treatment related toxicity [116, 117].

As mycophenolate mofetil is a rather cell selective immunosuppressant with potent activity on both activated T and B lymphocytes (and probably monocytes), while lacking the broad, nondiscriminant toxicity towards proliferating cells inherent in most alkylating agents and anti-metabolites, it is an attractive drug for treatment of (presumed) autoimmune diseases. Fueled by positive results in animal models [119–121], and anecdotal reports in transplant recipients with concomitant glomerulonephritis [122], cases and small series of results of mycophenolate mofetil treatment in various diseases such as autoimmune skin disorders [123–125], biliary disease [126], inflammatory bowel disease [127, 128], glomerular disease [129, 130], and lupus nephritis [131] have been reported.

Clinical data on mycophenolate mofetil therapy in primary vasculitis

Mycophenolate mofetil is mentioned as a very promising alternative to alkylating agents in the treatment of primary vasculitic syndromes in several reviews [132–134]. Firm data to claim and substantiate a role for mycophenolate mofetil in the standard treatment of primary vasculitis are as yet lacking. As is usually the case, new treatment options are first attempted in patients in which current standard therapy has proven ineffective or cannot be used. The limited data obtained so far, however, are promising. A recent report documented the successful treatment of active Takayasu's arteritis in three patients not responding to steroids and cytotoxic agents [135]. As especially in ANCA-related vasculitis such as Wegener's granulomatosis the need for less toxic therapies is high, cases with active disease refractory or intolerant to standard therapy with cyclophosphamide have been treated. Successful treatment in a patient with severe active Wegener's granulomatosis, intolerant to cyclophosphamide with mycophenolate mofetil combined with corticosteroids has been recently reported [136]. Some groups have reported on small series of patients with active ANCA-related vasculitis, either Wegener's granulomatosis or microscopic polyangiitis, treated with mycophenolate mofetil for different reasons [137–139]. In 13 of 20 patients with active vasculitis remission was achieved with mycophenolate mofetil 1 to 2 g/day in combination with corticosteroids, while four could not tolerate mycophenolate mofetil due to gastrointestinal side-effects and three did not respond. No serious hematological toxicity or serious opportunistic infections were encountered [137–139].

We have recently treated 13 patients with a relapse of ANCA positive Wegener's granulomatosis who were intolerant to cyclophosphamide with oral mycophenolate mofetil (2 g/day) in combination with prednisolone (0.5–1.0 mg/kg/day with successive tapering) [140]. Active glomerulonephritis at the moment of diagnosis of relapse was present in seven (in five cases proven by renal biopsy). Cyclophosphamide treatment was precluded due to hemorrhagic cystitis, locally treated bladder cancer, bone marrow failure, or relapse during maximal tolerated cyclophosphamide therapy. The majority of patients were on azathioprine maintenance therapy (1–2 mg/kg/day) in combination with low-dose corticosteroids at the moment of relapse. All patients responded to treatment with mycophenolate mofetil and prednisolone with complete and partial remission of disease activity in 11 and two patients, respectively. Relapses during treatment occurred in three patients after 5 to 10 months, while 10 are still in complete remission for a median of 14 months since the start of treatment with mycophenolate mofetil. Gastrointestinal side-effects and anaemia were observed in two patients each, all responding to reducing the mycophenolate mofetil dose. Otherwise therapy was well tolerated without serious infectious complications [140]. The limited data so far suggest that mycophenolate mofetil combined with corticosteroids is a viable option in the treatment of patients with active ANCA-related vasculitis unresponsive or intolerant to cyclophosphamide. In addition, mycophenolate mofetil in combination with low dose steroids has successfully been used for maintenance therapy in small series of patients following a relapse of ANCA-associated Wegener's granulomatosis and microscopic polyangiitis with renal involvement after remission was induced with cyclophosphamide [137, 141].

The future role of 15-deoxyspergualin and mycophenolate mofetil in treatment of primary vasculitic syndromes

The optimal place of 15-deoxyspergualin and mycohenolate mofetil in the therapeutic armamentarium for remission induction and maintenance therapy in primary vasculitis and especially the ANCA-related syndromes is currently unclear. Preliminary data available so far suggest that both 15-deoxyspergualin and mycophenolate mofetil can be of potential value in a range of situations. Whether these drugs are an adequate alternative or may even be superior to drugs like cyclophosphamide and methotrexate for induction therapy or azathioprine for maintenance therapy can only be answered by adequately powered, well-designed, controlled studies. These studies are, given the low incidence of primary vasculitic syndromes, only possible with extensive collaborative efforts by the patients and their treating physicians.

Acknowlegements
The authors are indepted to Nippon Kayaku Japan/Germany, particularly to Dr. J.M. Drexler, for providing confidential data concerning 15-deoxyspergualin. Moreover, the support from Dr. R. Nowack, Lindau, Germany, as well as the critical review of the manuscript by Prof. Dr. F.J. van der Woude, Mannheim, Germany, is appreciated.

References

1   Fauci AS, Haynes BF, Katz P (1978) The spectrum of vasculitis: clinical, pathologic, immunologic and therapeutic considerations. *Ann Intern Med* 89: 660–676

2   Jennette JC, Falk RJ, Andrassy K, Bacon PA, Churg J, Gross WL, Hagen EC, Hoffman GS, Hunder GG, Kallenberg CGM et al (1994) Nomenclature of systemic vasculitides. Proposal of an International Consensus Conference. *Arthritis Rheum* 37: 187–192

3   Kallenberg CGM, Brouwer E, Weening JJ, Cohen Tervaert JW (1994) Anti-neutrophil cytoplasmic antibodies: current diagnostic and pathophysiological potential. *Kidney Int* 46: 1–15

4   Evans J, Hunder GG (1998) Polymyalgia rheumatica and giant cell arteritis. *Clin Geriatr Med* 14: 455–473

5   Rai A, Nast C, Adler S (1999) Henoch-Schönlein purpura nephritis. *J Am Soc Nephrol* 10: 2637–2644

6   Guillevin L, Lhote F (1998) Treatment of polyarteritis nodosa and microscopic polyangiitis. *Arthritis Rheum* 41: 2100–2105

7   Guillevin L (1999) Treatment of classic polyarteritis nodosa in 1999. *Nephrol Dial Transplant* 14: 2077–2079

8   Leung DY, Schlievert PM, Meissner HC (1998) The immunopathogenesis of Kawasaki syndrome. *Arthritis Rheum* 41: 1538–1547

9   Laupland KB, Dele Davies H (1999) Epidemiology, etiology, and management of Kawasaki's disease. State of the art. *Pediatr Cardiol* 20: 177–183

10   Fauci AS, Katz P, Haynes BF, Wolff SM (1979) Cyclophosphamide therapy of severe systemic necrotizing vasculitis. *N Engl J Med* 301: 235–238

11   Fauci AS, Haynes BF, Katz P, Wolff SM (1983) Wegener's Granulomatosis: prospective clinical and therapeutic experience with 85 patients for 21 years. *Ann Intern Med* 98: 76–85

12   Jennette JC, Falk RJ (1997) Small-vessel vasculitis. *N Engl J Med* 337: 1512–1523

13   Hoffman GS, Kerr GS, Leavitt RY, Hallahan CW, Lebovics RS, Travis WD, Rottem M, Fauci AS (1992) Wegener's granulomatosis: an analysis of 158 patients. *Ann Intern Med* 116: 488–498

14   Gordon M, Luqmani RA, Adu D, Greaves I, Richards N, Michael J, Emery P, Howie AJ, Bacon PA (1993) Relapses in patients with a systemic vasculitis. *Q J Med* 86: 779–789

15   Boumpas DT, Austin HA, Vaughan EM, Yarboro CH, Klippel JH, Balow JE (1993) Risk for sustained amenorrhea in patients with systemic lupus erythematosus receiving intermittent pulse cyclophosphamide therapy. *Ann Intern Med* 119: 366–369

16   Masala A, Faedda R, Alagna S, Satta A, Chiarelli G, Rovasio PP, Ivaldi R, Taras MS, Lai E, Bartoli E (1997) Use of testosterone to prevent cyclophosphamide-induced azoospermia. *Ann Intern Med* 126: 292–295

17   Langford CA, Klippel JH, Balow JE, James SP, Sneller MC (1998) Use of cytotoxic agents and cyclosporine in the treatment of autoimmune disease. Part 2: Inflammatory bowel disease, systemic vasculitis, and therapeutic toxicity. *Ann Intern Med* 129: 49–58

18   Radis CD, Kahl LE, Baker GL, Wasko MC, Cash JM, Gallatin A, Stolzer BL, Agarwal AK, Medsger Jr TA, Kwoh CK (1995) Effects of cyclophosphamide on the development of malignancy and on long term survival of patients with rheumatoid arthritis. *Arthritis Rheum* 38: 1120–1127

19   Talar-Williams C, Hijazi YM, Walther MM, Linehan WM, Hallahan CW, Lubensky I, Kerr GS, Hoffman GS, Fauci AS, Sneller MC (1996) Cyclophosphamide-induced cystitis and bladder cancer in patients with Wegener's granulomatosis. *Ann Intern Med* 124: 477–484

20   Westman KWA, Bygren PG, Olsson H, Ranstam J, Wieslnader J (1998) Relapse rate, renal survival and cancer morbidity in patients with Wegener's granulomatosis or microscopic polyangiitis with renal involvement. *J Am Soc Nephrol* 9: 842–852

21   Adu D, Pall A, Luqmani RA, Richards NT, Howie AJ, Emery P, Michael J, Savage COS, Bacon P (1997) Controlled trial of pulse versus continuous prednisolone and cyclophosphamide in the treatment of systemic vasculitis. *Q J Med* 90: 401–409

22   Guillevin L, Cordier JF, Lhote F, Cohen P, Jarrousse B, Royer I, Lesavre Ph, Jacquot C, Bindi P, Bielefeld P et al (1997) A prospective, multicenter, randomized trial comparing steroids and pulse cyclophosphamide in the treatment of generalized Wegener's granulomatosis. *Arthritis Rheum* 40: 2187–2198

23   Haubitz M, Schellong S, Göbel U, Schurek HJ, Schaumann D, Koch KM, Brunkhorst R (1998) Intravenous pulse administration of cyclophosphamide versus daily oral treatment in patients with antineutrophil cytoplasmic antibody-associated vasculitis and renal involvement. A prospective, randomized study. *Arthritis Rheum* 41: 1835–1844

24   de Groot K, Adu D, Savage COS (2000) To pulse or not to pulse in ANCA-associated vasculitis – a critical analysis. *Clin Exp Immunol* 120 (Suppl 1): 68

25   Sneller MC, Hoffman GS, Talar-Williams C, Kerr GS, Hallahan CW, Fauci AS (1995) An analysis of forty-two Wegener's granulomatosis patients treated with methotrexate and prednisone. *Arthritis Rheum* 38: 608–613

26   De Groot K, Mühler M, Reinhold-Keller E, Paulsen J, Gross WL (1998) Induction of

remission in Wegener's granulomatosis with low dose methotrexate. *J Rheumatol* 25: 492–495

27 Stone JH, Tun W, Hellman DB (1999) Treatment of non-life threatening Wegener's granulomatosis with methotrexate and daily prednisone as the initial therapy of choice. *J Rheumatol* 26: 1134–1139

28 Reinhold-Keller E, de Groot K, Rudert H, Nölle B, Heller M, Gross WL (1996) Response to trimethoprim/sulfamethoxazole in Wegener's granulomatosis depends on the phase of the disease. *Q J Med* 89: 15–23

29 Jayne DRW, Gaskin G (EUVAS) (1999) Randomised trial of cyclophosphamide versus azathioprine during remission in ANCA-associated vasculitis (CYCAZAREM). *J Am Soc Nephrol* 10: 105A

30 de Groot K, Reinhold-Keller E, Tatsis E, Paulsen J, Heller M, Gross WL (1996) Therapy for maintenace of remission in sixty-five patients with generalized Wegener's granulomatosis. Methotrexate versus trimethoprim-sulfamethoxazole. *Arthritis Rheum* 39: 2052–2061

31 Haubitz M, Koch KM, Brunkhorst R (1998) Cyclosporin for the prevention of disease reactivation in relapsing ANCA-associated vasculitis. *Nephrol Dial Transplant* 13: 2074–2076

32 Stegeman CA, Cohen Tervaert JW, de Jong PE, Kallenberg CGM (1996) Trimethoprim-sulfamethoxazole for the prevention of relapses of Wegener's granulomatosis. *N Engl J Med* 335: 16–20

33 Pedersen RS, Bistrup C (1996) Etoposide: more effective and less bone-marrow toxic than standard immunosuppressive therapy in systemc vasculitis? *Nephrol Dial Transplant* 11: 1121–1123

34 Takeuchi T, Linuma H, Kunimoto S, Masuda T, Ishizuka M, Takeuchi M, Hamada M, Naganawa H, Kondo S, Umezawa H (1981) A new antitumor antibiotic, spergualin: Isolation and antitumor activity. *J Antibiot* 34: 1619

35 Maeda K, Umeda Y, Saino T (1993) Synthesis and background chemistry of 15-deoxyspergualin. *Ann NY Acad Sci* 685: 123–135

36 Nishikawa K, Shibasaki C, Takahashi K, Nakamura T, Takeuchi T, Umezawa H (1986) Antitumor activity of spergualin: a novel antitumor antibiotic. *J Antibiot* 39: 1461–1466

37 Muindi JF, Lee SJ, Baltzer L, Jakubowski A, Scher HI, Sprancmanis LA, Riley CM, Vander Velde D, Young CW (1991) Clinical pharmacology of deoxyspergualin in patients with advanced cancer. *Cancer Res* 12: 3096

38 Thies J, Walter P, Zimmermann F, Dickneite G, Sedlacek H, Keller H, Feifel G (1987) Prolongation of graft survival in allogenic pancreas and liver transplantation by 15-deoxyspergualin. *Eur Surg Res* 19: 129–134

39 Dickneite G, Schorlemmer H, Weinmann E, Bartlett R, Sedlacek H (1987) Skin transplantation in rats and monkeys: Evaluation of efficient treatment with 15-deoxyspergualin. *Transplant Proc* 19: 4244–4247

40 Reichenspurner H, Hildebrandt A, Human PA, Boehm DH, Rose AG, Odell JA,

Reichart B, Schorlemmer H (1990) 15-Deoxyspergualin for induction of graft nonreactivity after cardiac and renal allotransplantation in primates. *Transplantation* 50: 181–185

41   Engemann R, Gassell HJ, Lafrenz E, Stoffregen C, Thiede A (1987) Transplantation tolerance after short-term administration of 15-deoxyspergualin in orthotopic rat liver transplantation. *Transplant Proc* 19: 4241–4243

42   Fukao K, Otsuka M, Iwashaki H, Yuzawa K, Iwasaki Y (1989) Immunosuppressive effect of deoxyspergualin on acute renal allograft rejection in dogs. *Transplant Proc* 21: 1090–1093

43   Nicolic-Patterson DJ, Kerr PG, Lan HY, Tesch GH, Atkins RC. Deoxyspergualin: A new immunosuppressive drug for the treatment of auto-immune disease. *Nephron* 1995; 70: 391–396

44   Fujii H, Takada T, Nemoto K, Yamashita T, Abe F, Fujii F, Takeuchi T (1990) Deoxyspergualin directly suppresses antibody formation *in vivo* and *in vitro*. *J Antibiot* 43: 213–219

45   Makino M, Fujiwara M, Watanabe H, Aoyagi T, Umezawa H (1987) Immunosuppressive activities of deoxyspergualin. II. The effect of the antibody responses. *Immunopharmacol* 14: 115–122

46   Tepper MA, Petty B, Bursuker I, Pasternak RD, Cleaveland J, Spitalny GL, Schacter B Inhibition of antibody production by the immunosuppressive agent, 15-deoxyspergualin. *Transplant Proc* 23: 328–331

47   Tepper M, Nadler S, Mazzucco C, Singh C, Kelley S (1993) Mechanism of action of 15-deoxyspergualin, a novel immunosuppressive drug. *Ann NY Acad Sci* 685: 122–135

48   Investigation Report Form of the Results of Use to the Ministry of Health and Welfare, Nippon Kayaku Co. Ltd., 1998

49   Fujii H, Takada H, Kyuichi T, Fuminori N, Fujii A, Talmadge A, Takeuchi J (1992) Deoxyspergualin, a novel immunosuppressant, markedly inhibits human mixed lymphocyte reaction and cytotoxic T-lymphocyte activation *in vitro*. *Int J Immunopharmacol* 14: 731–737

50   Odaka C, Toyoda E, Nemoto K (1998) Immunosuppressant deoxyspergualin induces apoptotic cell death in dividing cells. *Immunology* 95: 370–376

51   Morikowa K, Oseko F, Moridawa S (1992) The suppressive effect of deoxyspergualin on the differentiation of human B lymphocytes maturating into immunoglobulin-producing cells. *Transplantation* 54: 526–531

52   Sterbenz KG, Tepper MA (1994) The effect of 15-deoxyspergualin on antibody secretion from antibody producing B-cell hybridomas and myelomas. *Transplant Proc* 26: 3218

53   Tepper MA, Nadler SG, Esselstyn J, Sterbenz C (1995) Deoxyspergualin inhibits kappa light chain expression in 70Z/3 pre-B cells by blocking lipopolysaccharide induced NF-kappaB activation. *J Immunol* 155: 2427–2436

54   Wang B, Benoist C, Mathis D (1996) The immunosuppressant 15-deoxyspergualin

reveals commonality between PreT and PreB cell differentiation. *J Exp Med* 183: 2427–2436

55 Dickneite G, Schorlemmer HU, Sedlacek HH (1987) Decrease of mononuclear phago-cyte cell functions and prolongation of graft survival in experimental transplantation by 15-deoxyspergualin. *Int J Immunopharmacol* 9: 559–565

56 Takasu S, Sakagami K, Morisaki F, Kawamura T, Haisa M, Oiwa T, Inagaki M, Hasuo-ka H, Kurozumi Y, Orita K (1991) Immunosuppressive mechanism of 15-deoxysper-gualin on sinusoidal lining cells in swine liver transplantation: suppression of MHC class II antigens and interleukin-1 production. *J Surg Res* 51: 165–169

57 Kerr PG, Nikolic-Paterson DJ, Lan HY, Rainone S, Tesch G, Atkins RC (1994) Deoxyspergualin suppresses local macrophage proliferation in renal allograft rejection. *Transplantation* 58: 596–601

58 Hoeger P, Tepper MA, Faith A, Higgins J, Lamb J, Geha R (1994) The immunosup-pressant deoxyspergualin inhibits antigen processing in monocyts. *J Immunol* 153: 3908–3916

59 Nadler SG, Tepper MA, Schacter B, Mazzucco CE (1994) Interaction of the immuno-suppressant deoxyspergualin with a member of the HSP 70 family of heat shock pro-teins. *Science* 258: 484–486

60 Nadeau K, Nadler SG, Saulnier M, Tepper MA, Walsh CT (1994) Quantitation of the interaction of the immunosuppressant deoxyspergualin and analogs with Hsc70 and Hsp90. *Biochemistry* 33: 2561–2567

61 Smith DV, Whitesell L, Katsanis E (1998) Molecular chaperones: Biology and prospects for pharmacological intervention. *Pharmacol Rev* 4: 493–513

62 DeNagel DC, Pierce SK (1993) Heat shock proteins in immune responses. *Crit Rev Immunol* 13: 71–81

63 Tepper MA (1996) *In vitro* pharmacology, mechanism of action and preclinical phar-macokinetics and toxicology of DSG. In: R Lieberman, A Mukherjee (eds): *Principles of drug development in transplantation and autoimmunity*. RG Landes Company, London, 383–388

64 Gore PF (1996) Deoxyspergualin: clinical experience. *Transplant Proc* 2: 871–872

65 Ohlman S, Zilg H, Schindel F, Lindholm A (1994) Pharmacokinetics of 15-deoxysper-gualin studied in renal transplant patients receiving the drug during graft rejection. *Transpl Int* 1: 5–10

66 Pilot study phase I study of gusperimus in rheumatoid arthritis, Bristol-Myers Squibb Pharmaceutical Research Institute, 1995

67 Pilot study phase I study of gusperimus in multiple sclerosis, Bristol-Myers Squibb Phar-maceutical Research Institute, 1993

68 Comparison of pharmacokinetics in Caucasians and Japanese, Behringwerke AG, 1993

69 Havlin KA, Kuhn JG, Koeller J, Boldt DH, Craig JB, Brown TD, Weiss GR, Cagnola J, Phillips J, Harman G et al (1995) Deoxyspergualin: phase I clinical, immunologic and pharmacokinetic study. *Anticancer Drugs* 2: 229–236

141

70   Ronneberger H (1994) Pharmacological-toxicological expert opinion on immodul. Behringwerke AG

71   Ramos EL, Nadler SG, Grasela DM, Kelley SL (1996) Deoxyspergualin: mechanism of action and pharmacokinetics. *Transplant Proc* 2: 873–875

72   Ohlman S, Zilg H, Schindel F, Lindholm A (1994) Pharmacokinetics of 15-deoxyspergualin studied in renal transplant patients receiving the drug during graft rejection. *Transplant Int* 7:5–10

73   Single dose safety, tolerance and pharmacokinetics of subcutaneous administration of gusperimus in healthy subjects, Bristol-Myers Squibb Pharmaceutical Research Institute, 1994

74   Phase I study of subcutaneous gusperimus in patients with rheumatoid arthritis, Bristol-Myers Squibb Pharmaceutical Research Institute, 1996

75   Micronucleus test using mice treated with NKT-01 (N40), June 29, 1987, report of Nippon Kayaku, Japan

76   Intravenous micronucleus study in rats, Bristol-Myers Squibb Pharmaceutical Research Institute, 1994

77   Mutagenicity study of NKT-01 using microorganisms, Sogo Biomedical Laboratories, 1986

78   Chromosome aberration study of NKT-01 using mammal cultivated cells, Sogo Biomedical Laboratories, 1986

79   *In vitro* mammalian cytogenetic test in cultured human lymphocytes, CIT, 1993

80   Ames reverse-mutation study in *Salmonella* and *Escherichia coli*, Bristol-Myers Squibb Pharmaceutical Research Institute,1993

81   Ames/*Salmonella* microbial mutagenicity study including *Escherichia coli* WP2 uvrA, Bristol-Myers Squibb Pharmaceutical Research Institute, 1993

82   Chromosome aberration study in cultured mammalian (CHL) cells, Bristol-Myers Squibb Pharmaceutical Research Institute,1993

83   Cytogenetics study in primary human lymphocytes, Bristol-Myers Squibb Pharmaceutical Research Institute,1993

84   The effect of i.v. injection of NKT-01 on rats during the period of fetal organogenesis (segment II), Nihon Bioresearch center, 1986

85   Teratogenicity study of NKT-01 in rabbits (intravenous administration), Nippon Kayaku, 1991

86   Segment II intravenous teratology study in rats with an evaluation of postnatal development, Bristol-Myers Squibb Pharmaceutical Research Institute,1993

87   Segment II intravenous teratology study in rabbits, Bristol-Myers Squibb Pharmaceutical Research Institute,1993

88   Segment III intravenous perinatal/postnatal study in rats, Bristol-Myers Squibb Pharmaceutical Research Institute, 1993

89   One-year intraperitoneal toxicity study in rats with a nine-week recovery period, Bristol-Myers Squibb Pharmaceutical Research Institute, 1993

90 Prospective, placebo-controlled, randomized, double-blind multicentre Phase III in patients suffering from multiple sclerosis, Behringwerke AG, 1996

91 Thomas FT, Tepper MA, Thomas JM, Haisch CE (1993) 15-Deoxyspergualin: a novel immunosuppressive drug with clinical potential. *Ann NY Acad Sci* 685: 172–195

92 Okubo M, Tamura K, Kamata K, Tsukamoto Y, Nakayama Y, Osakabe T, Sato K, Go M, Kumano K, Endo T (1993) 15-deoxyspergualin "rescue therapy" for methylpred-nisolone-resistant rejection of renal transplants as compared with anti-T cell monoclonal antibody (OKT3). *Transplantation* 55: 505–508

93 Miura s, Okazaki H, Sato T, Amada N, Sakurada M (1997) Succeful renal transplantation in presensitized recipients with double-filtration plasmapheresis and 15-deoxyspergualin. *Transplant Proc* 29: 350–351

94 Takahashi K, Yagisawa T, Sonda K, Kawaguchi Y, Yamaguchi H, Toma H, Agishi T, Ota K (1993) ABO-incompatible kidney transplantation in a single-center trial. *Transplant Proc* 1: 271–273

95 Groth CG, Ohlman S, Ericzon BG, Barkholt L, Reinholt FP (1990) Deoxyspergualin for liver graft rejection. *Lancet* 336: 626

96 Dhingra K, Fritsche H, Murray JL, LoBuglio AF, Khazaeli MB, Kelley S, Tepper MA, Grasela D, Buzdar A, Valero V et al (1995) Phase I clinical and pharmacological study of suppression of human antimouse antibody response to monoclonal antibody L6 by deoxyspergualin. *Cancer Res* 14: 3030–3067

97 Birck R, Nowack R, Drexler JM, Hotta O, Goebel, van der Woude FJ (1999) 15-Deoxyspergualin induces remission in Wegener's Granulomatosis: report of three cases. [Abstract] *J Am Soc Nephrol* 11: 154A

98 Hotta O, Ito K, Furuta T, Chiba S, Taguma Y (1999) Effects of deoxyspergualin on proliferative glomerulonephritis. *Nippon Jinzo Gakkai Shi* 1:21–8

99 Nelson P, Eugui E, Allison AC (1990) Synthesis and immunosuppressive activity of some side- chain variants of mycophenolic acid. *J Med Chem* 33: 833–838

100 Lee W, Gu L, Miksztal AR, Chu N, Leung K, Nelson PH (1990) Bioavailability improvement of mycophenolic acid through amino ester derivatization. *Pharm Res* 7: 161–166.

101 Eugui EM, Alquist SJ, Muller CD, Allison AC (1991) Lymphocyte-selective cytostatic and immunosuppressive effects of mycophenolic acid *in vitro*: role of deoxyguanosine nucleotide depletion. *Scand J Immunol* 33: 161–173

102 Allison AC, Eugui EM (1996) Purine metabolism and immunosuppressive effects of mycophenolate mofetil (MMF). *Clin Transplant* 10: 77–84

103 Allison AC, Eugui EM (1993). Immunosuppressive and other effects of mycophenolic acid and ester prodrug, mycophenolate mofetil. *Immunol Rev* 136: 5–28

104 Natsumeda Y, Carr SF (1993). Human type I and type II IMP dehydrogenase as targets. *Ann NY Acad Sci* 696: 88–93

105 Dayton J, Lindsten T, Thompsom CB, Mitchell BS (1994) Effects of human T lymphocyte activation on inosine monophosphate dehydrogenase expression. *J Immunol* 52: 984–991

106 Bullingham R, Monroe S, Nicholls A, Hale M (1996) Pharmacokinetics and bioavail-

ability of mycophenolate mofetil in healthy subjects after single-dose oral and intravenous administration. *J Clin Pharmacol* 36: 315–324

107 Bullingham RES, Nicholls A, Hale M (1996) Pharmacokinetics of mycophenolate mofetil (RS 61443): a short review. *Transplant Proc* 28: 925–929

108 Sham LM, Nowak I (1995) Mycophenolic acid: measurement and relationship to pharmacological effects. *Ther Drug Monit* 17: 690–699

109 Lipsky JJ (1996) Mycophenolate mofetil. *Lancet* 348: 1357–1359

110 Nowak I, Shaw LM (1995) Mycophenolic acid binding to human serum albumin: characterization and relation to pharmacodynamics. *Clin Chem* 41: 1011–1017

111 Kaplan B, Gruber SA, Nallamathou R, Katz SM, Shaw LM (1998) Decreased protein binding of mycophenolic acid associated with leukopenia in a pancreas transplant recipient with renal failure. *Transplantation* 65: 1127–1129

112 Epinette WW, Parker CM, Jones EL, Greist MC (1987) Mycophenolic acid for psoriasis. *J Am Acad Dermatol* 17: 962–971

113 European Mycophenolate Mofetil Cooperative Study Group (1995) Placebo-controlled study of mycophenolate mofetil combined with cyclosporin and corticosteroids for prevention of acute rejection. *Lancet* 345: 1321–1325

114 Sollinger HW for the U.S. Renal Transplant Mycophenolate Mofetil Study Group (1995) Mycophenolate mofetil for the prevention of acute rejection in primary cadaveric renal allograft recipients. *Transplantation* 60: 225–232.

115 Tricontinental Mycophenolate Mofetil Renal Transplant Study Group (1996) A blinded, randomized clinical trial of mycophenolate mofetil for the prevention of acute rejection in cadaveric renal transplantation. *Transplantation* 61: 1029–1037

116 Halloran P, Mathew T, Tomlanovich S, Groth C, Hooftman L, Barker C, for the International Mycophenolate Mofetil Renal Transplant Study Groups (1997) Mycophenolate mofetil in renal allograft recipients. A pooled efficacy analysis of three randomized, double-blind, clinical studies in prevention of rejection. *Transplantation* 63: 39–47

117 Mathew T, for the Tricontinental Mycophenolate Mofetil Renal Transplant Study Group (1998) A blinded, long-term, randomized multicenter study of mycophenolate mofetil in cadaveric renal transplantation. Results at three years. *Transplantation* 65: 1450–1454

118 Kim YS, Moon JI, Kim SI, Park K (1999) Clear benefit of mycophenolate mofetil-based triple therapy in reducing the incidence of acute rejection after living donor renal transplantation. *Transplantation* 68: 578–581

119 Van Bruggen MCJ, Walgreen B, Rijke TPM, Berden JHM (1998) Attenuation of murine lupus nephritis by mycophenolate mofetil. *J Am Soc Nephrol* 9: 1407–1415

120 Jonsson CA, Svensson L, Carlsten H (1999) Beneficial effect of the inosine monophosphate dehydrogenase inhibitor mycophenolate mofetil on survival and severity of glomerulonephritis in systemic lupus erythematosus (SLE)-prone MRLlpr/lpr mice. *Clin Exp Immunol* 116: 534–541

121 Remuzzi G, Zoja C, Gagliardini E, Corna D, Abbate M, Benigni A (1999) Combining

an antiproteinuric approach with mycophenolate mofetil fully suppresses progressive nephropathy of experimental animals. *J Am Soc Nephrol* 10: 1542–1549

122 Adams PL, Iskandar SS, Rohr MS (1999) Biopsy-proven resolution of immune complex-mediated crescentic glomerulonephritis with mycophenolate mofetil therapy in an allograft. *Am J Kidney Dis* 33: 552–554

123 Nousari HC, Sragovich A, Kimyai-Asadi A, Orlinsky D, Anhalt GJ (1999) Mycophenolate mofetil in autoimmune and inflammatory skin disorders. *J Am Acad Dermatol* 40: 265–268

124 Enk AH, Knop J (1999) Mycophenolate is effective in the treatment of pemphigus vulgaris. *Arch Dermatol* 135: 54–56

125 Grundmann-Kollmann M, Kaskel P, Leiter U, Krahn G, Ralf S, Peter U, Kerscher M (1999) treatment of pemphigus vulgaris and bullous pemphigoid with mycophenolate mofetil monotherapy. *Arch Dermatol* 135: 724–725

126 Altschuler EL (1999) Mycophenolate mofetil for primary biliary cirrhosis and sclerosing cholangitis? *Nephrol Dial Transplant* 14: 798–799

127 Neurath MF, Wanitschke R, Peters M, Krummenauer F, Zum Buschenfelde K-HM, Schlaak JF (1999) Randomised trial of mycophenolate mofetil versus azathioprine for treatment of chronic active Crohn's disease. *Gut* 44: 625–628

128 Present DH (1999) Is mycophenolate mofetil a new alternative in the treatment of inflammatory bowel disease? *Gut* 44: 592–593

129 Nowack R, Birck R, van der Woude FJ (1997) Mycophenolate mofetil for systemic vasculitis and IgA nephropathy. *Lancet* 349: 774

130 Briggs WA, Choi MJ, Scheel PJ Jr, Kiberd B, MacDonald A (1998) Successful mycophenolate mofetil treatment of glomerular disease. *Am J Kidney Dis* 31: 213–217

131 Dooley MA, Cosio FG, Nachman PH, Falkenhain ME, Hogan SL, Falk RJ, Hebert LA (1999) Mycophenolate mofetil therapy in lupus nephritis: clinical observations. *J Am Soc Nephrol* 10: 833–839

132 Hauser IA, Sterzel RB (1999) Mycophenolate mofetil: therapeutic applications in kidney transplantation and immune-mediated renal disease. *Curr Opin Nephrol Hypertens* 8: 1–6

133 Gross WL (1999) New concepts in treatment protocols for severe systemic vasculitis. *Curr Opin Rheumatol* 11: 41–46

134 Jayne DRW (1999) Non-transplant uses of mycophenolate mofetil. *Curr Opin Nephrol Hypertens* 8: 563–567

135 Daina E, Schieppati A, Remuzzi G (1999) Mycophenolate mofetil for the treatment of Takayashu arteritis: report of three cases. *Ann Intern Med* 130: 422–426

136 Waiser J, Budde K, Braasch E, Neumayer HH (1999) Treatment of c-ANCA-positive vasculitis with mycophenolate mofetil. *Am J Kidney Dis* 34: e9 (www.ajkd.org)

137 Haidinger M, Neumann I, Jäger H, Grützmacher H, Bayer P, Meisl FTh (2000) Mycophenolate mofetil treatment of ANCA-associated small-vessel vasculitis: a pharmacokinetically controlled study. *Clin Exp Immunol* 120 (Suppl 1): 72

138 Nachman PH, Joy MS, Hogan SL, Jennette JC, Falk RJ (2000) Mycophenolate mofetil:

preliminary results of a feasibility trial in relapsing ANCA small vessel vasculitis. *Clin Exp Immunol* 120 (Suppl.1): 72

139 Pesavento TE, Falkenhain ME, Rovin BH, Hebert LA (1999) Mycophenolate mofetil in anti-neutrophil cytoplasmic antibody vasculitis. *J Am Soc Nephrol* 10: 114A

140 Stegeman CA, Cohen Tervaert JW (2000) Mycophenolate mofetil for remission induction in patients with active Wegener's granulomatosis intolerant to cyclophosphamide. *J Am Soc Nephrol* 11: 98A

141 Nowack R, Göbel U, Klooker P, Hergesell O, Andrassy K, van der Woude FJ (1999) Mycophenolate mofetil for maintenance therapy of Wegener's granulomatosis and microscopic polyangiitis: a pilot study in 11 patients with renal involvement. *J Am Soc Nephrol* 10: 1965–1971

Interferon-α for the treatment of virus-related systemic vasculitides

Loïc Guillevin

Department of Internal Medicine, Université Paris-Nord, Hôpital Avicenne, Assistance Publique – Hôpitaux de Paris, 125, rue de Stalingrad, 93009 Bobigny cedex, France

Introduction

Interferon-α (IFNα) is now widely used to treat virus-associated vasculitides. This treatment is based on different mechanisms and is indicated for different purposes: (1) a specific antiviral treatment in virus-related vasculitides; (2) an immunomodulating therapy specifically or non-specifically targeting the vasculitic process and not its etiology; (3) a treatment that reduces liver fibrosis progression [1]. Only IFNα has been prescribed for vasculitis and we will concentrate in this chapter on its indication in virus-related vasculitides: polyarteritis nodosa (PAN) related to hepatitis B virus (HBV) and cryoglobulinemia as the consequence of hepatitis C virus (HCV) infection. We will not comment here on the treatment of non-viral vasculitides with IFNα. Two types of IFNα are commonly prescribed, IFNα 2a and IFNα 2b. They differ by one amino acid but no difference in efficacy has been shown. The other types of IFN, that is, IFNβ and IFNγ, are not prescribed for virus-associated vasculitides.

Interferon therapy in virus-associated vasculitis

Treatment of HBV-related PAN

Main characteristics of HBV-related PAN
The main clinical and biological characteristics of HBV-related PAN have been extensively described elsewhere [2] and we focus here only on some points which will facilitate the understanding of the therapeutic section. Without any ambiguities, HBV-related PAN should be considered as a strict form of classical PAN. The clinical manifestations fit perfectly with the American College of Rheumatology (ACR) classification criteria for PAN [3] and with the Chapel Hill Nomenclature [4]. When nephropathy is present, it is exclusively ischemic with a typical angiogram showing multiple microaneurysms, stenoses and renal infarcts. This vascular nephropathy explains the high frequency of severe and malignant hypertension [5]. Orchitis is

Disease-modifying Therapy in Vasculitides, edited by Cees G. M. Kallenberg and
Jan W. Cohen Tervaert
© 2001 Birkhäuser Verlag Basel/Switzerland

also a frequent symptom, observed in 26% of patients [2]. With a well-adapted treatment the outcome is now better than in the past when patients were treated with cyclophosphamide and steroids [6]. The 7-year survival rate is 83% and relapses are infrequent. In a long-term study [7] concentrating on the outcome of PAN, microscopic polyangiitis and Churg-Strauss syndrome, we observed that only 7.9% of the patients relapsed, a rate significantly lower than in other vasculitides. This explains why this "one-shot" disease might best be treated with a short and intensive therapeutic regimen focused on the etiology and acute manifestations of the disease, without continuing with a maintenance treatment which seems unnecessary.

HBV-PAN is an acute post-infectious disease that occurs within 6 to 18 months after infection, in case this point in time can be determined. Vasculitis rarely develops after or concomitantly with acute hepatitis. Hepatitis is asymptomatic and jaundice extremely rare. Hepatic cytolysis is mild and transaminases are two to four times above the normal range, rarely more. Liver biopsy can be normal or show the presence of subacute or chronic hepatitis. Liver biopsy rarely demonstrates vasculitis.

Treatment

For many years, HBV-related PAN was treated in the same way as non-virus-related PAN, and patients received steroids, sometimes combined with cytotoxic agents, mainly cyclophosphamide. This treatment was often effective in the short-term, but careful analysis of long-term results showed the occurrence of relapses and complications related to viral persistence resulting in chronic hepatitis or liver cirrhosis. In the paper by McMahon et al. [8], in which PAN was observed in Eskimos, four patients (31%) died during the course of PAN. In our first randomized study [9] in which patients were not selected according to their viral status, 14 out of 71 patients with PAN were HBV positive; 84% of them recovered from PAN but two subsequently died of liver cirrhosis. Antiviral drugs were prescribed for viral hepatitis and showed their effectiveness.

In 1988 [10, 11] in conjunction with Christian Trépo who described HBV as underlying the development of PAN [12], we decided to treat HBV-related PAN with a combination of antiviral treatment and plasma exchanges, after short-term steroid treatment. An abrupt stopping of steroids or cytotoxic agents was essential for the efficacy of antiviral treatment, because steroids and other immunosuppressants stimulate virus replication. An alternative therapy was also needed to reduce the mortality of PAN and to improve prognosis. In a retrospective study, we showed that when steroids and immunosuppressants were prescribed to HBV-related PAN, the outcome was poorer than in non viral-PAN [6].

Based on the efficacy of antiviral agents in chronic hepatitis [13] and of plasma exchange in PAN, we combined both therapies to treat HBV-related PAN. The rationale of the therapeutic approach was as follows: initially corticosteroids to rapidly control the most severe life-threatening manifestations of PAN which are common during the first weeks of the disease, and then abrupt discontinuation to enhance immunological clearance of HBV-infected hepatocytes and favor seroconversion of HBe antigen (Ag) positivity to anti-HBe antibody (Ab) positivity; during this phase plasma exchange to control the course of PAN.

When this therapeutic strategy was first applied, the only available antiviral agent was vidarabine. 33 patients were treated, 24 newly diagnosed patients and nine who had failed to respond to steroids and cytotoxic agents. After a 3-week course of vidarabine, administered after 1 week of steroids (1 mg/kg/day) combined with plasma exchange, a full clinical recovery was obtained in three-quarters of the patients and HBe Ag to anti-HBe Ab seroconversion was observed in nearly half of the patients. HBs Ag to anti-HBs Ab seroconversion was obtained in 18% of the group only. This low rate of seroconversion was attributed to the limited efficacy of vidarabine and by early integration of the viral genome into hepatocytes.

Interferon-α

In an attempt to improve therapeutic outcome, vidarabine was replaced by IFNα. IFNα is a powerful agent, against both DNA and RNA viruses. It is the recommended treatment for HBV hepatitis and has been shown to be effective. Practically, IFN offers the advantage to be administered subcutaneously and, therefore, a shorter hospital stay can be expected. Among the first six patients included in the study [14], seroconversion of HBeAg to anti-HBeAb was observed in four patients (66.7%) and that of HBsAg to anti-HBsAb in 3/6 (50%). The treatment has now been extended to 12 patients (unpublished data) and the initial seroconversion rate has been confirmed. One patient died of infectious side-effects (septicemia via an indwelling catheter). IFNα should therefore be recommended as the first-line treatment for HBV-related PAN. Also on the long term, treatment was effective and relapses were rare, 5.6% [2].

The dose of IFNα is comparable to that prescribed for hepatitis B, i.e., 3 million units, three times a week. When no seroconversion is observed, the dose can be increased to 6 million units, three times a week. Treatment is, in fact, better tolerated than expected. During the first days of administration, fever, myalgias, malaise and fatigue may occur. They are usually transient and disappear over the following weeks. The simultaneous administration of paracetamol is recommended. The long-term side effects of IFNα include hypothyroidism, which was never observed in our patients, mainly because the duration of the prescription did not exceed 6 months for the majority of patients. In only rare cases, it was necessary to administer IFNα for more than 1 year in order to obtain seroconversion, even though PAN had been cured for several months.

Although this approach appears suitable, it has not been confirmed in a randomized study comparing this pathophysiological strategy to conventional treatment. Nevertheless, it is not reasonable to propose such a trial in light of the good results obtained under antiviral therapy which is also able to cure PAN in a few weeks. In addition, the efficacy of this approach has been confirmed by others who treated patients with IFNα alone [15, 18]. IFNα has also been combined with famciclovir [16] or lamivudine, another powerful drug against DNA viruses [17].

Plasma exchanges

In a few cases [15, 18] the antiviral agent was prescribed alone. In our opinion, even if it is possible to obtain good clinical results in some patients, the severity of the disease in most patients requires therapy able to immediately control the severe or life-threatening manifestations of PAN. Plasma exchanges are able to rapidly clear the immune complexes responsible for the disease. This rapid intervention is most appropriate to control the disease. In our protocol, steroids are also prescribed for a few days at the start of treatment to control the clinical manifestations as quickly as possible while waiting for the effect of IFNα. In our opinion, plasma exchange is not indicated because of its superiority to other regimens, but because it is in combination with antiviral drugs equivalent in efficacy to other deleterious therapies that are commonly used in virus-associated vasculitides.

The optimal schedule of plasma exchange is as follows: four sessions/week for 3 weeks, then three sessions/week for 2 to 3 weeks, followed by tapering of the frequency of plasma exchange. One plasma volume (60 ml/kg) is usually exchanged using 4% albumin replacement fluid. The circuit can be primed with starch. During the first weeks of treatment the high number of plasma exchanges can decrease the level of clotting factors and thereby lead to bleeding. Should bleeding occur, fresh frozen plasma can be used instead of albumin as replacement fluid. Usually, PE is excellently tolerated, although some of our patients have experienced minor side-effects [19].

The simultaneous use of plasma exchange on the one hand and vidarabine or IFNα on the other could clear the latter drugs more rapidly. We examined this possibility for vidarabine [20] and demonstrated that, even when vidarabine was administered simultaneously with plasmapheresis, only a minor amount of the drug was cleared, and thus no extra drug supplementation was required. Because subcutaneously administered IFNα is generally given in the evening following plasma exchange, measurement of serum IFNα levels does not seem necessary. This was not the case for intravenous IFNα treatment, which was prescribed to treat cryoglobulinemia (see below).

Outcome and follow-up

The short- and long-term outcomes of the patients have been previously described and showed progressive improvement of seroconversion rates for patients receiving IFNα. We can expect that new antiviral therapies and novel drug combinations will bring further improvement in terms of definitive suppression of the virus. One of the major advances obtained under this antiviral strategy was the very rapid cure of PAN, even in its most severe forms. The majority of patients received the antiviral drug for a few weeks or months and plasma exchange, which was specifically given to control the acute manifestations of the disease, was stopped after 2 months. It was sometimes possible to eliminate all signs of vasculitis even more quickly, with patients recovering within 3 weeks.

In the days following treatment onset, transaminase levels decreased. They usually returned to normal within a few days or weeks. When patients were treated with vidarabine, a second increase of transaminase levels was observed prior to seroconversion. This immunological response was considered normal and reflected the patient's ability to attack the virus within the hepatocytes. This response was usually mild and expected in the patients as it confirmed the recovery from the disease. Nevertheless, an enhanced response can occur and fulminant hepatitis can be observed simultaneously with seroconversion, as was the case in one of our patients [21] who died of fulminant hepatitis in the days following HBe/anti HBe seroconversion. The response observed on IFNα is markedly different. Levels of transaminase normalize insidiously and there is no rebound in their level after stopping treatment, even when seroconversion has not been obtained.

When antibodies directed against the virus are detected, plasmapheresis should be stopped in order to avoid the clearance of the newly synthesized antibodies. In a few cases, levels of antibodies fluctuated, sometimes being present and sometimes absent. In the latter case treatment should be continued. In such cases, it is more reliable to monitor viral load by quantitative measurements of viral DNA.

After recovery from the symptoms of the disease, the clinician potentially faces two different virological situations. First, replication is still present, as demonstrated by the absence of HBe Ab and by the positivity of viral DNA. Although remission of PAN has been obtained relapses may then still occur. We therefore recommend continuing IFNα administration to 6 or 12 months according to the viral response as measured by quantitative viral DNA assessment and to focus on treatment of viral hepatitis and not on PAN which is in remission. Second, antibodies to HBe, at least, or to HBs, at best, are present and the patient can be considered cured. Relapses will never occur. If, despite the presence of antibodies to HBs, new manifestations of PAN develop, the clinician should consider the possibility that vasculitis occurred coincidentally with HBV infection but was not linked to it.

Treatment of HCV cryoglobulinemia

Clinical characteristics of HCV-related cryoglobulinemia
Mixed cryoglobulinemia of type II and more rarely type III are the consequence

of HCV infection in more than 80% of the patients [22]. Cryoglobulinemia is asymptomatic in most patients but persists for decades. Disease duration is associated with the occurrence of clinical symptoms, not always coinciding with the onset of cryoglobulinemia. When symptoms are present, the most frequent symptoms are purpura, peripheral neuropathy, glomerulonephritis, leg ulcers, arthritis and sicca syndrome. Relapses are usual, and the disease is chronic even under treatment.

Treatment: general principles

Only 15 to 20% of the patients with chronic hepatitis C achieve a sustained virological response [23]. For the majority of cases, no treatment is able to cure mixed cryoglobulinemia definitively and the therapeutic strategy has not yet been clearly defined. Steroids and immunosuppressive drugs are commonly used to treat severe forms, but they stimulate virus replication and can accelerate the development of chronic hepatitis and cirrhosis, conditions which facilitate the occurrence of liver cancer. We therefore devised a strategy comprising antiviral drugs and plasma exchange for some patients [24]. In asymptomatic patients, there is no argument to treat, and monitoring could be sufficient. In patients with moderate symptoms (arthralgias, purpura, sensory peripheral neuropathy, for instance), IFNα alone or in combination with ribavirin should be tested. The probability to sustain long-term disappearance of the virus and cryoglobulinemia remains low, less than 25% of patients, despite good initial responses [24, 25].

Interferon-α and other antiviral agents

Treating cryoglobulinemia with IFNα is based on the regimen prescribed for HCV hepatitis, a disease in which half of the patients are found to have more-or-less asymptomatic cryoglobulinemia, when it is systematically looked for. We also know, from extensive experience with hepatitis, that virological results are poor [23] and that the virus remains present in approximately 80% of the patients. Mixed cryoglobulinemia with clinical symptoms seems to be a disease that develops after a decades-long chronic infection, and, although there are no data to support a correlation between the time of infection and disease activity, we hypothesize that it is more difficult to obtain viral clearance and recovery from the disease during the chronic phase of cryoglobulinemia.

Clinical prospective trials using IFNα alone [25], or in combination with plasma exchange and/or low-dose steroids [24] showed that the majority of patients improved clinically on treatment and that the viral replication rate decreased in the majority of the patients [24], but that a relapse occurred in 83% of the patients immediately after stopping treatment. In prospective trials [24, 25] patients were treated for 6 months only, which is obviously insufficient to obtain satisfactory results. This period was, however, the recommended treatment duration for hepatitis at the time of the studies on cryoglobulinemia, and no new prospective trials have been proposed in this field for the last 5 years. However, this unsatisfactory result could be accepted if the disease was clinically controlled and liver function improved. Maintenance therapy could be proposed with prolonged IFNα administration at the same or lower dose in order to "control" disease progression and clinical symptoms, while waiting for more effective treatment regimen that are able to clear the virus and to cure cryoglobulinemia.

At present, combining two antiviral drugs, IFNα and ribavirin is indicated. Ribavirin alone is not able to completely suppress viral replication but, in conjunction with IFNα, viral replication was no longer detectable in 48% of the patients [23] receiving this combination for 12 months. We can expect that suppression of viral replication can also be obtained in cryoglobulinemia.

A correlation between viral load and cryoglobulinemia also needs to be confirmed. Although the majority of the patients seen for symptomatic cryoglobulinemia have virus-positive polymerase chain reactions (PCR), reflecting viral replication, a few of them remain serologically positive but become PCR negative, reflecting past contamination. We also observed, in two of our patients who presented with very severe vasculitis, disappearance of the virus under antiviral treatment and plasma exchange, but persistence of clinical symptoms necessitating a prolonged symptomatic treatment with plasma exchange.

In order to be more effective against the virus, we recently tried to treat patients with intravenous IFNα. The rationale for this treatment was based on the expected effect of sequential treatment on hepatocyte receptors for the virus. IFNα was infused at a dose of 1 million units/m^2, every 12 h. The dose was adapted every week to the virological response. The dose can be increased by 0.5 million units/m^2 up to a maximum dose of 2.5 million units/m^2 every 12 h. Once the optimal dose able to induce the disappearance of the virus as measured by PCR was obtained, IFNα was administered for another 4 to 5 weeks. In case of side-effects, for example moderate thrombocytopenia or renal insufficiency, the IFNα dose can be lowered or IFNα withdrawn. Only three patients were treated and treatment had to be stopped because of side-effects: one patient developed atrial arrhythmia and all of them experienced intense fatigue with myalgias and fever. The treatment was definitively stopped when thrombocytopenia occurred in one of these three patients. This latter side-effect is not rare in this disease because patients simultaneously present chronic liver hepatitis or cirrhosis and portal hypertension with hypersplenism. Nevertheless, the virological results were excellent, with lower PCR values being obtained in all the patients in the first hours after starting the infusion. Complete suppression of viral replication was observed in 1/3 patients, by 5 weeks of treatment. Unfortunately, sustained suppression was never obtained, and viral replication increased rapidly several days after stopping intravenous IFNα despite subcutaneous maintenance therapy (three million units, three times a week).

The results obtained with IFNα emphasize the need for more powerful agents, or antiviral combinations, to combat HCV infection.

Plasma exchange

The indication for plasma exchange in HCV-related cryoglobulinemia is controversial. We recommend the combination of plasma exchange and antiviral drugs based on the effectiveness observed in our patients who failed to respond to other treatments and on the publication of several failures of IFNα to have an effect on severe mixed cryoglobulinemia [26]. Plasma exchange should not be prescribed systematically for every newly diagnosed case of cryoglobulinemia because the majority of patients present no or very few symptoms, and we do not know at present whether or not treatment is indeed indicated in these pauci- or asymptomatic forms of cryoglobulinemia. Plasma exchange is indicated for patients with symptoms requiring medical intervention. Purpura and sicca syndrome are not indications for plasmapheresis: the former regresses spontaneously and the latter is refractory to this treatment. In the case of glomerulonephritis due to cryoglobulinemia, plasma exchange combined with IFNα can be effective, but randomized controlled trials are needed to assess their contribution. Plasma exchange is mainly indicated to treat rapidly progressive peripheral neuropathy and leg ulcers. The latter manifestation is often very severe and accompanied with pain that can require intensive treatments, including morphine. Under plasma exchange, arteriolar ulcers regress quickly and complete healing can be obtained in a few weeks. Plasma exchange should be tapered slowly to avoid a rebound phenomenon due to the increased production of cryoglobulins as a consequence of the stimulation of the B-cell clone responsible for their production. Several patients remain plasma exchange-dependent: clinical symptoms re-occur or worsen while tapering or after abrupt discontinuation of the sessions. Maintenance treatment should therefore be prescribed and the clinician has to try to determine the minimal number of sessions able to control the disease.

The number of sessions is, however, not clearly established. We propose the following schedule: three sessions a week for 3 weeks, then two sessions a week for 2 to 3 weeks, then one session every week or every 10 days until clinical symptoms disappear or the optimal clinical result is obtained. Adjuvant treatment remains mandatory to avoid or reduce the intensity of the rebound phenomenon.

The technical aspects of plasmapheresis are of major importance. Conventional plasma exchange is performed by centrifugation or filtration and the same principles as described above for HBV-PAN are applied. In addition, the extracorporal circuit should be heated to avoid precipitation of cryoglobulins. Immunoadsorption is not recommended at present due to the risk of precipitation of the cryoglobulins in the column. New advances in this field would probably enable the use of this technique, which offers the advantage of clearing more globulins than conventional plasmapheresis.

Other treatments

Chronic treatment is frequently prescribed for mixed cryoglobulinemia. Steroids and/or immunosuppressive drugs are indicated for severe cases which do not respond to IFNα and plasma exchange. They are prescribed as a last resort because no other option exists. They are effective on clinical symptoms and the patient improves. Long-term treatment is more problematic and liver function should be carefully monitored.

Interferon-induced side effects

In rare cases, IFNα has been described as being responsible for vasculitis [27], in cases where it had been prescribed for viral hepatitis. A putative relationship between IFNα treatment and the development of vasculitis was postulated. Nevertheless, unlike autoimmune diseases that can exacerbate under IFNα treatment [28], the occurrence of vasculitis remains rare and should not limit IFNα use when it is indicated.

Conclusion

IFNα is now part of the standard treatment of virus-associated vasculitis and should be prescribed in stead of steroids and cytotoxic agents. This therapeutic approach, whether or not with plasma exchange, is logical and adapted to the etiology of the disease. Although its superiority has been demonstrated in prospective studies [2, 24, 25], its limitations are also obvious, and IFNα alone is not able to cure the majority of the patients. The combination of several antiviral agents, or new antiviral drugs will probably improve patients' outcome. It is also probable that plasma exchange will remain a major part of the therapeutic regimen. Technological improvements and the development of immunoadsorption could accelerate patient recovery.

References

1   Poynard T (1997) Interferon alpha in hepatitis C: a cytokine for reducing fibrosis progression. *Eur Cytokine Netw* 8: 319–320
2   Guillevin L, Lhote F, Cohen P, Sauvaget F, Jarrousse B, Lortholary O, Noel LH, Trépo C (1995) Polyarteritis nodosa related to hepatitis B virus. A prospective study with long-term observation of 41 patients. *Medicine (Baltimore)* 74: 238–253
3   Lightfoot RJ, Michel BA, Bloch DA, Hunder GG, Zvaifler NJ, McShane DJ, Arend WP,

Calabrese LH, Leavitt RY, Lie JT et al (1990) The American College of Rheumatology 1990 criteria for the classification of polyarteritis nodosa. *Arthritis Rheum* 33: 1088–1093

4   Jennette JC, Falk RJ, Andrassy K, Bacon PA, Churg J, Gross WL, Hagen EC, Hoffman GS, Hunder GG, Kallenberg CG et al (1994) Nomenclature of systemic vasculitides. Proposal of an international consensus conference. *Arthritis Rheum* 37: 187–192

5   Cohen L, Guillevin L, Meyrier A, Bironne P, Blétry O, Godeau P (1986) Hypertension artérielle maligne au cours de la périartérite noueuse. Incidence, paramètres clinico-biologiques et pronostic chez 165 patients. *Arch Mal Coeur Vaiss* 79: 773–778

6   Guillevin L, Lê T, Gayraud M (1989) Systemic vasculitis of the polyarteritis nodosa group and infection with hepatitis B virus: a study in 98 patients. *Eur J Intern Med* 1: 97–105

7   Gayraud M, Guillevin L, Le Toumelin P, Cohen P, Lhote F, Casassus P, Jarrousse B (2001) Long-term follow-up of polyarteritis nodosa, micropolyangiitis and Churg-Strauss syndrome: analysis of 4 prospective trials including 278 patients. *Arthritis Rheum* 44: 666–675

8   McMahon BJ, Heyward WL, Templin DW, Clement D, Lanier AP (1989) Hepatitis B-associated polyarteritis nodosa in Alaskan Eskimos: clinical and epidemiologic features and long-term follow-up. *Hepatology* 9: 97–101

9   Guillevin L, Jarrousse B, Lok C, Lhote F, Jais JP, Le Thi Huong Du, Bussel A (1991) Longterm followup after treatment of polyarteritis nodosa and Churg-Strauss angiitis with comparison of steroids, plasma exchange and cyclophosphamide to steroids and plasma exchange. A prospective randomized trial of 71 patients. The Cooperative Study Group for Polyarteritis Nodosa. *J Rheumatol* 18: 567–574

10   Guillevin L, Merrouche Y, Gayraud M (1988) Périartérite noueuse liée au virus de l'hépatite B. Détermination d'une stratégie thérapeutique nouvelle: 13 observations. *Presse Med* 17: 1522–1526

11   Trépo C, Ouzan D, Delmont J, Tremisi P (1988) Supériorité d'un nouveau traitement curateur des périartérites noueueses induites par le virus de l'hépatite B grâce à l'association corticothérapie brève, vidarabine et échanges plasmatiques. *Presse Méd* 17: 1527–1531

12   Trépo C, Thivolet J (1970) Antigen Australia, hépatite à virus et périartérite noueuse. *Presse Méd* 78: 1575

13   Lok A, Novack D, Karahiannis P, Dunk A, Sherlock S, Thomas H (1985) A randomized study of the effects of adenine arabinoside 5'-monophosphate (short or long course) and lymphoblastoid interferon on hepatitis B virus replication. *Hepatology* 5: 1132–1138

14   Guillevin L, Lhote F, Sauvaget F, Deblois P, Rossi F, Levallois D, Pourrat J, Christoforov B, Trépo C et al (1994) Treatment of polyarteritis nodosa related to hepatitis B virus with interferon-alpha and plasma exchanges. *Ann Rheum Dis* 53: 334–337

15   Avsar E, Savas B, Tözün N, Ulusoy NB, Kalayci C (1998) Successful treatment of polyarteritis nodosa related to hepatitis B virus with interferon alpha as first-line therapy [letter]. *J Hepatol* 28: 525–526

16 Kruger M, Böker KH, Zeidler H, Manns MP (1997) Treatment of hepatitis B-related polyarteritis nodosa with famciclovir and interferon alfa-2b. *J Hepatol* 26: 935–939

17 Wicki J, Olivieri J, Pizzolato G, Sarasin F, Guillevin L, Dayer JM, Chizzolini C (1999) Successful treatment of polyarteritis nodosa related to hepatitis B virus with a combination of lamivudine and interferon alpha [letter]. *Rheumatology (Oxford)* 38: 183–185

18 Simsek H, Telatar H (1995) Successful treatment of hepatitis B virus-associated polyarteritis nodosa by interferon alpha alone. *J Clin Gastroenterol* 20: 263–265

19 Lhote F, Guillevin L, Bussel A, Léon A, Lok C, Toledano D, Sobel A, Baudelot J (1987) Side effects of therapeutic plasma exchange during treatment of polyarteritis nodosa. Comparison of filtration and centrifugation: 718 sessions in 63 patients. *Life Support Syst* 5: 359–366

20 Fauvelle F, Leon A, Nicolas P, Tod M, Guillevin L, Petitjean O (1992) Pharmacokinetics of vidarabine in the treatment of polyarteritis nodosa. *Fundam Clin Pharmacol* 6: 11–15

21 Guillevin L, Lhote F, Léon A, Fauvelle F, Vivitski L, Trépo C (1993) Treatment of polyarteritis nodosa related to hepatitis B virus with short-term steroid therapy associated with antiviral agents and plasma exchanges. A prospective trial in 33 patients. *J Rheumatol* 20: 289–298

22 Agnello V, Chung RT, Kaplan LM (1992) A role for hepatitis C virus infection in type II cryoglobulinemia. *N Engl J Med* 327: 1490–1495

23 Poynard T, Marcellin P, Lee S, Niederau C, Minuk GS, Ideo G, Bain V, Heathcote J, Zeuzeri S, Trépo C et al (1998) Randomized trial of interferon alpha2b plus ribavirin for 48 weeks or for 24 weeks versus interferon alpha 2b plus placebo for 48 weeks for treatment of chronic infection with hepatitis C virus. International Hepatitis Interventional Therapy Group. *Lancet* 352: 1426–1432

24 Cohen P, Nguyen QT, Deny P, Ferrière F, Roulot D, Lortholary O, Jarrousse B, Danon F, Barrier JH, Ceccaldi J et al (1996) Treatment of mixed cryoglobulinemia with recombinant interferon alpha and adjuvant therapies. *Ann Méd Intern (Paris)* 147: 81–86

25 Ferri C, Marzo E, Longbardo G (1993) Interferon-alpha in mixed cryoglobulinemia patients. A randomized crossover-controlled trial. *Blood* 81: 1132–1136

26 Roithinger FX, Allinger S, Kirchgatterer A, Prischl F, Balon R, Haidenthaler A, Knoflach P (1995) A lethal course of chronic hepatitis C, glomerulonephritis, and pulmonary vasculitis unresponsive to interferon treatment. *Am J Gastroenterol* 90: 1006–1008

27 Pateron D, Fain O, Sehonnou J, Trinchet JC, Beaugrand M (1996) Severe necrotizing vasculitis in a patient with hepatitis C virus infection treated by interferon. *Clin Exp Rheumatol* 14: 79–81

28 Conlon K, Urba W, Smith J, Steis R, Longo D, Clark J (1990) Exacerbation of symptoms of autoimmune disease in patients receiving alpha-interferon therapy. *Cancer* 65: 2237–2242

Autologous stem cell therapy for systemic vasculitis

David M. Carruthers[1] and Paul A. Bacon[2]

[1]Department of Rheumatology, City Hospital NHS Trust, Dudley Road, Birmingham B18 7QH, UK; [2]Department of Rheumatology, Division of Immunity and Infection, University of Birmingham, Edgbaston, Birmingham B15 2TT, England

Introduction

Stem cell transplantation (SCT) has been proposed as a potentially highly effective therapy for a variety of autoimmune diseases. In this group of diseases a disturbed immune response results in an attack by the immune system on host antigens with B- and T-cell components involved in the process. The hypothesis behind SCT in autoimmune disease is that a vigorous immuno-ablative preparation regimen ("conditioning") can delete the patient's immune system with subsequent haemo- and lymphopoietic reconstitution from infused pluripotent progenitor stem cells (SC). Success would thus require that both pathogenic auto-aggressive T-cell clones are deleted from the host and that the triggering "environmental" factor be no longer present once the immune system is reconstituted from SC precursors. Such triggers may be particularly likely to persist, or be produced by the local inflammatory microenvironment. Alternatively, the newly developed immune system may develop tolerance to the antigenic trigger allowing an effective cure of the autoimmune disease. However, more simply, a third explanation is that prolonged remission is induced through immune response modulation secondary to the intensive conditioning immunosuppression.

In this chapter we will discuss the rationale behind, approaches to and issues surrounding the possible mechanisms of action of high dose immunosuppression followed by SCT. Many of the questions that have arisen from the use of this procedure in autoimmune disease and their probable relevance in systemic necrotizing vasculitis (SNV) will be highlighted. Firstly, however, we will consider the reasons for suggesting that SNV patients may present potentially suitable candidates for such therapy.

Disease-modifying Therapy in Vasculitides, edited by Cees G. M. Kallenberg and
Jan W. Cohen Tervaert
© 2001 Birkhäuser Verlag Basel/Switzerland

Rationale for stem cell transplantation in systemic vasculitis

Immunological abnormalities in systemic vasculitis

Several pathogenic mechanisms and cell types contribute to vessel damage in SNV, but exactly how the inflammatory process is initiated or perpetuated is unknown. Endothelial cells, which form the barrier between the blood stream and vessel wall, play a critical role [1]. Immune complexes (IC) and anti-endothelial antibodies may be involved in initiation of the disease, with IC deposition in the vessel wall activating complement and attracting neutrophils *via* chemotactic factors. Necrotizing vasculitis ensues with thrombosis, occlusion, haemorrhage and secondary ischaemia of local tissues. Endothelial damage is also induced by activated neutrophils which infiltrate and degranulate at the vessel wall. These neutrophils may have been primed by low levels of circulating pro-inflammatory cytokines which can arise secondary to local infection. Further activation of primed neutrophils by IgG anti-neutrophil cytoplasmic antibody (ANCA) results in the release of lytic enzymes and reactive oxygen species, products which induce inflammation in the vessel wall at the sites of neutrophil adhesion [2].

In addition, there is increasing evidence for the role of the T cell in the pathogenesis of vasculitis. This is particularly well documented in giant cell arteritis where there is evidence of a local antigen driven process [3]. In ANCA-related vasculitis there may be T-cell reactivity against either the vessel wall or antigenic components of proteinase 3 (PR3) and myeloperoxidase (MPO) which have been released from activated neutrophils and become adherent to the endothelium [4]. There is also evidence of a Th1 pattern of cytokine production from peripheral blood (PB) T cells in active Wegener's granulomatosis (WG), perhaps promoting a cell mediated response in this disease [5]. However, the precise role played by the T cell in the production of ANCA, anti-endothelial antibodies and destructive granuloma in WG is unclear. Thus, in SNV there is a complicated interaction between activated neutrophils, T and B cells and the endothelium. The effects of cyclophosphamide (Cy) on each of these cell types may be critical for its therapeutic effect, making it the most appropriate drug for use both as standard therapy and as part of a conditioning protocol prior to SCT in patients with SNV.

Cyclophosphamide therapy for systemic vasculitis

Cyclophosphamide is the most effective drug for the therapy of SNV, with arguments now focusing on not whether, but how best to use it. The 5-year survival of patients treated with Cy is now 80%, transforming the prognosis of SNV from diseases with high acute mortality to chronic relapsing diseases with high morbidity [6,

7]. Although remission is induced in greater than 90% of patients, the response to continuous oral Cy (2 mg/kg/day) is often slow with up to 2 years Cy therapy needed in some cases and relapse occurring in almost 50% of patients [8]. In this large study, these factors combined to give a total disease free period of less than half the patient months of follow-up, increasing the need for prolonged courses of Cy and therefore an increased risk of drug toxicity. When the cumulative dose of Cy is > 100 g, the risk of serious bladder problems, including cancer, are clearly unacceptable [9]. In addition, a slow response to therapy causes early morbidity and long-term complications secondary to serious tissue damage. In one controlled trial standard pulse Cy regimens (15 mg/kg/pulse) did not reduce disease activity scores any faster than continuous oral Cy (2 mg/kg/day) but pulse therapy may have been associated with less toxicity [10]. An early response to therapy with complete suppression of disease activity would be ideal, reducing both the need for prolonged Cy therapy to induce remission and the risk of organ damage that occurs secondary to grumbling disease activity. This damage accrues maximally during the 6 months after first presentation [11] and thus the first flare of disease is the ideal time to attempt to reduce long-term problems by early remission induction.

High-dose cyclophosphamide therapy for systemic vasculitis

We proposed that more intense immunosuppression for a flare of disease activity would be beneficial, reducing the morbidity that results from accumulation of items of organ damage. Using oncological data from the therapy of haematological malignancy [12, 13] we devised short, high-dose pulse Cy regimens that were given for 3 months only and delivered the same total dose of Cy as is given with 3 months daily oral Cy (~ 14 gms). Doses of Cy which were up to four times the size of individual standard Cy pulses were given in our new high-dose protocols. Six pulses were given at 3 weekly intervals, either as two cycles of three pulses in descending doses (maximum dose 2.5 g/m^2), or as six equal size pulses (1.4 g/m^2) (Carruthers et al., submitted). Remission was induced rapidly, achieving a reduction in the validated disease activity score, BVAS [14], to zero by 2 months in nine out of 13 patients treated, a rate of response not seen in any other published series [10]. In some instances neutropenia (< 1 × 10^9/l) occurred after the highest doses of Cy and this may partly explain the good early response seen with these high-dose protocols as neutrophils are intimately involved in the inflammatory vascular lesions. Relapse following remission induction, even during the series of six pulses, was common and may have been driven by infection that occurred in association with the severe immunosuppression. We have since modified the pulses to diminish the infection risk. However, this limited study does provide proof of concept that disease activity can be rapidly suppressed in SNV by intensive immunosuppression.

High-dose cyclophosphamide in therapy of autoimmune disease

Others have used high-dose chemotherapy without SC rescue for the therapy of rheumatoid arthritis (RA) and aplastic anaemia. When intensified dose Cy (4 g/m^2) was used for SC mobilisation for two RA patients who had associated scleritis and rheumatoid vasculitis there was complete and persistent clearance of these extra-articular manifestations, but the synovitis, though improved initially, later relapsed [15]. In seven out of 10 patients with aplastic anaemia an apparent cure was achieved with 180 mg/kg Cy given over 4 days [16]. Here it was proposed that the immuno-ablative high dose Cy may have destroyed auto-aggressive lymphocyte clones that were driving the autoimmune disease and a *de novo* regenerating immune system did not remember the antigenic properties of previous clones. The same group have applied a similar approach to 11 patients with SLE where 200 mg/kg Cy was given without SC rescue [17]. These patients had all previously failed conventional immunosuppressive therapy and they were able to achieve complete remission in five of them with this high-dose approach. As SC are resistant to high-dose Cy they argue that SCT is unnecessary as BM recovery will occur and in fact lessens the chance of disease relapse as there is no infusion of potentially autoreactive T cells. Their longest follow-up was 20 months, so we will have to wait and see if prolonged remission can be induced with Cy alone. A critical feature when aiming for such prolonged remissions in autoimmune disease relates to the effect of Cy on host lymphocyte populations.

Effects of cyclophosphamide on the immune system

Cyclophosphamide is a pro-drug for one or more bifunctional alkylating agents with phosphoramide mustard being the most biologically active product after oxidative activation. Cells may be acted on at any stage of the cell cycle, but most of the effect occurs when the cell enters S phase with progression through the cell cycle blocked at G2. The amount of DNA alkylation is a function of the dose of drug administered, with the likelihood of cell death related to the degree of alkylation. Rapidly dividing cell populations such as hair follicles, gastrointestinal epithelium and bone marrow are most affected. High-dose pulse Cy induces a fall in platelet count with recovery occurring after 3 weeks while neutropenia is induced 7–10 days after administration, with full recovery generally also occurring by day 21. This neutropenia, which is related to the dose of Cy given and is presumably secondary to acute cell death, may confer a beneficial response in SNV. During flares of activity in SNV there is significant neutrophil infiltration in the vessel wall and surrounding tissues, the extent of which has been associated with the degree of disease activity [18], and is likely to contribute to organ damage. Rapid elimination of these cells may enhance the rate of remission induction and reduce the morbidity and damage that occurs during prolonged flares of disease activity.

Both continuous oral and bolus Cy produce a depression in circulating B- and T-cell numbers. It appears that mature (memory) cell populations, compared with naïve cells, are less sensitive to continuous low dose oral Cy than they are to high dose pulse Cy [19]. If SNV are antigen driven diseases, then for an effective cure it will be important to delete the circulating memory T cells that are driving the disease process. Therefore, as memory T cells are more resistant to conventional doses of immuno-suppressants, high-dose chemotherapy, chemo-radiation or other lympholytic agents may be required for complete ablation of anti-self reactive immune T cells. If this can be achieved then newly developing lymphocytes from uncommitted progenitor cells may be re-educated, with the hope that they acquire tolerance to self antigens [20] or come more effectively under control by peripheral tolerance mechanisms.

If such intense immunosuppression is given that all bone marrow derivatives, including activated neutrophils and auto-aggressive T-cell clones are deleted then a "cure" in SNV, or at least long-term clinical remission, is feasible provided that marrow recovery is possible. As Cy appears to have a SC sparing effect, irreversible marrow aplasia after boluses as high as 250 mg/kg rarely occurs, but there is often a long delay until full marrow recovery [12]. In this situation, and specially if additional myeloablative therapy is given, SC rescue with previous harvested cells is likely to be necessary to repopulate the marrow and hasten the regeneration of a functioning immune system.

Approach to stem cell transplantation

Haemopoietic stem cells

Haemopoietic SCs are bone marrow (BM) cells that are capable of self renewal and differentiation, leading to the production of all cells of the immune system. Common lymphoid and myeloid progenitors as well as erythroblasts and megakaryocytes are derived in the marrow from this rare pluripotent population of cells (Fig. 1). Human SC, thought to reside in a small fraction (1–3%) of the BM cells that express the CD34 antigen, lead to long-term marrow recovery after SCT. However, more developmentally restricted progenitor cells which are already primed to undergo rapid proliferation and development lead to recovery in the short term. These CD34+ SCs can be obtained either directly from the BM or from the peripheral blood (PB) after appropriate mobilisation regimens with colony stimulating factors (CSF) alone or in combination with chemotherapy. A theoretical advantage in using SCs obtained directly from BM in the therapy of autoimmune diseases is that the graft will contain fewer T cells, which include potentially autoreactive ones.

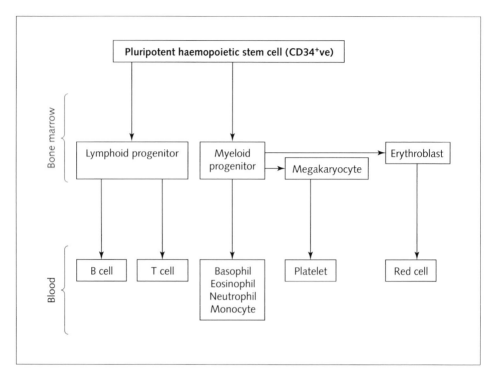

Figure 1.
Development of CD34+ stem cells

However, peripheral SC harvest has several practical advantages. In particular it is a far simpler and more comfortable procedure for the patient. SC harvested from PB after mobilisation regimens contain a higher number of committed progenitor cells leading to a faster and more complete haemopoietic recovery in the host, especially of platelets. This beneficial effect can be combined with purification of harvested donor SC to remove mature T cells thus reducing the risk of relapse.

Donor SC used to repopulate the marrow may be syngeneic (identical twin), allogeneic (HLA identical sibling) or autologous (SC harvested from the individual who is to receive the transplant at a later date). Much of the early experience of SCT in patients with autoimmune disease came from allogeneic transplants needed primarily to treat associated malignancy. However, mortality from complications related to allogeneic transplant is high (15–35%) [21], mainly from graft *versus* host disease (GVHD). The use of autologous SC for marrow re-population, where transplant related mortality is < 3% [22], has become the recommended choice for therapy directed at autoimmune disease [21].

Stem cell mobilisation regimens

The SC mobilisation regimens used in the treatment of autoimmune diseases do not differ from those used for the therapy of haemopoietic malignancy. Mobilisation of SC into the PB for subsequent harvesting involves the use of either subcutaneous G-CSF (10 µg/kg/day) alone or in combination with pulse Cy (< 4 g/m^2), which is followed by G-CSF. There is a rapid increase in functionally normal neutrophils after G-CSF administration [23].

After mobilisation therapy, the number of CD34$^+$ cells in the PB is used as a surrogate marker for the optimal time for PB SC harvest. To achieve an adequate harvest of CD34$^+$ SC, three to four apharesis sessions are generally required after the circulating white cell count is $> 1 \times 10^9$/l. However, a single dose of Cy (4 g/m^2) can increase the number of circulating CFU-GM by 14-fold, thus reducing the number of apharesis sessions needed. A target SC dose for reinfusion into the host is $\geq 2.5 \times 10^6$ CD34$^+$ cells/kg, however if the graft is to be manipulated *ex vivo*, then $> 3 \times 10^6$ CD34$^+$/kg need to be harvested [21]. With these levels of PBSC, the reconstitution of haematopoiesis is very likely, though long-term studies are needed as there are some reports of incomplete engraftment and a slow recovery of the platelet count [24].

In patients who have had high cumulative doses of Cy for previous episodes of disease activity, SC mobilisation may be limited by marrow hypofunction, necessitating repeated SC harvests after further mobilisation therapy [25]. We have confirmed the ability to mobilise stem cells in two SNV patients despite such previous therapy. Also, we have harvested adequate numbers of CD34$^+$ PBSC from two other SNV patients after they had received 2.5 g/m^2 Cy (+ G-CSF) as part of our high-dose protocols for active disease. Colony stimulating factors, used in five of our SNV patients, have not resulted in a flare in disease activity, contrary to the situation in RA where recurrence of synovitis has been reported after its use [26].

Mobilisation with G-CSF without prior Cy can produce a good yield of SCs, but this may not be an appropriate approach in patients with SNV where the disease is likely to be active when SCT is considered. In this situation high-dose pulse Cy will have a dual role in the acute suppression of disease activity and SC mobilisation. Our experience with the high-dose pulse Cy regimens demonstrated proof of concept that remission in SNV could be induced rapidly with a more aggressive approach, albeit at an increased risk of early relapse. On this basis it is possible that remission may be induced in SNV after a single SC mobilisation regimen, although appropriate maintenance therapy is likely to be required. However, in one WG patient who was treated with high dose Cy, an excellent early clinical response for over 3 months was followed by a relapse. This flare in disease was controlled by full conditioning therapy and SCT.

Graft enrichment

One of the major theoretical limitations of PBSCT for autoimmune disease is that infusion of non-manipulated PBSC grafts allows the potential for re-infusion of a large number of immune cells, including autoreactive T cells which may restart the disease process. Therefore we believe that it is important to purify the SC before their re-infusion. Manipulation should aim to reduce the number of T cells within the graft to $< 1 \times 10^5$ cells/kg body weight [21, 27]. Such SC enrichment can be done using positive selection in a column where CD34$^+$ cells are bound by monoclonal antibodies linked to either microbeads or biotin, but there can be a significant loss of CD34 cells in the process requiring a larger initial SC harvest. Graft enrichment is an expensive, labour intensive process that is only worth doing if the conditioning therapy is sufficiently intensive to prevent regeneration of the aberrant immune system by residual cellular effectors. However, there is a risk of generating low grade immunodeficiency which increases the risk of infection and death, but it does have greater potential to suppress the autoimmune disease.

Conditioning regimens

The goal of applying high-dose chemotherapy prior to PBSCT in autoimmune disease is for the elimination of host immune lymphocytes, not tumour cells or host stem cells, so that only lymphocytotoxic agents such as Cy ± anti-lymphocyte antibodies ± total body irradiation (TBI) are indicated for conditioning. A variety of regimens have been proposed which include (i) Cy 50 gm/kg for 4 days ± anti-thymocyte globulin (ATG), (ii) Cy 60 mg/kg for 2 days + TBI, (iii) Busulphan 16 mg/kg over 4 days + Cy 60 mg/kg for 2 days, (iv) combination chemotherapy, BEAM (carmustine, etoposide, cytarabine, melphalan) [21].

It is unclear which myeloablative regimen achieves more complete immunoablation, including deletion of resting memory cells. Busulphan is also a bifunctional alkylating agent which is myeloablative at high doses, inducing prolonged suppression of CFU and granulocyte and macrophage precursors. It is therefore an anti-stem cell agent without immediate immunosuppressive properties and thus combines well with Cy. Anti-thymocyte globulin, with Cy, may be a more successful approach as it has immediate lytic effects on mature lymphocytes producing profound lymphopenia within 24 h of infusion, with recovery of the lymphocyte count by 1–3 weeks. It is therefore frequently used post PBSC infusion, in order to purge the T cells in the preparation (*in vivo* SC purging), and is a potential alternative to SC selection *ex vivo*. Total body irradiation is lympholytic and very effective at clearing progenitor cells but it is generally considered too risky to use in patients with autoimmune disease, although TBI has previously been utilised directly for the therapy of RA [28].

Effect of stem cell reconstitution on the immune system

The role of thymic dependent and independent T-cell regeneration

The aim of myelo-ablation and autologous PBSC graft enrichment is to allow generation of a new T-cell repertoire from the SC *via* the thymus. However, the ability of the thymus to regenerate T cells in adults after chemo or radiotherapy is in doubt and peripheral expansion of either T cells infused with the graft or the existing T-cell repertoire in the host may account for the major increase in T-cell number after SCT [29, 30]. Profound immuno-deficiency may therefore develop in adult patients with a poorly active thymus who have received high-dose T-cell ablative chemotherapy with a highly purified PBSC graft [31]. An upper age limit of 40 years for SCT is usually proposed for this reason.

Thymic independent regeneration of BM progenitors can occur in the gut, BM and liver but significant expansion of pre-existing mature T-cell populations can also occur in the periphery. This latter process is antigen driven so that most T cells will be recently activated and very few will be naïve. If there is a diverse antigen milieu in the host, T cells with a wide T-cell receptor Vβ family diversity and multiple specificities are generated. However, in the presence of limited antigenic stimulation a reduced expansion of the full TCR repertoire occurs with Vβ family skewing [29, 32, 33]. This results in decreased complexity of the T-cell compartment which has been correlated with the level of host immuno-competence [34, 35].

Immune reconstitution after stem cell therapy

After SCT, reconstitution of the myelomonocytic, megakaryocytic and erythroid lineages are directly related to the number of CD34+ cells in the graft [34], and in general the numbers of white cells, red cells and platelets are near normal 100 days after an allogeneic SCT [36–38]. However, as discussed above, the contribution of the SC graft to lymphoid engraftment is less clear and there are several factors which may contribute to a delay in immune reconstitution (Tab. 1) [39]. Functional reconstitution will occur if adequate maturation of lymphoid progenitors and pluripotent SCs into antigen specific T and B cells occurs within thymic and BM compartments [34], or if adequate numbers of antigen specific T and B cells remain in the graft or host after conditioning therapy [34, 38].

The phenotypic composition of the reformed T-cell population is also altered. There is a more rapid reconstitution of CD8+ than CD4+ T cells, leading to an inverted CD4/CD8 ratio in PB that approaches normal by 12 months [36, 38]. In addition, early (within 2 months) after SCT there is a high frequency of T cells expressing the memory CD45RO+ phenotype, but later the percentage of naïve, CD45RA T cells increases [34]. This suggests that the increase in circulating T cells

Table 1 - Reasons for delayed immunological reconstitution

Inverted CD4/CD8 ratio
Decreased NK cell activity
Decreased *in vivo* and *in vitro* cell mediated immunity
Decreased production and response to IL2
Decreased *in vivo* and *in vitro* antibody response to T-cell dependent antigen
Decreased T-cell Vβ repertoire

in the early period after SCT is due to the proliferation of either mature T cells that were present in the graft or residual T-cell populations in the host that were not eliminated by the conditioning therapy. T cells that appear later may be from SC that differentiated either in the residual thymus or at an extra thymic site of T-cell development during the post transplant period [34].

When functional responses are examined, T-cell proliferation is lower for up to 12 months in the recipients of T-cell depleted grafts, after which time proliferation equals those receiving conventional BMT [38]. This early functional impairment may be associated with an increase in infectious complications in the post transplant period [37].

Therefore, thymic function is limiting in adults and thymic independent pathways are probably insufficient for restoring full host immunocompetence. When considering PBSCT for autoimmune disease, a balance needs to exist between depletion of the autoaggressive T cells from both the graft and the host and the risk of severe immunodeficiency that will occur secondary to poor T-cell reconstitution.

Stem cell transplantation in autoimmune disease

Several animal models have shown prolonged remission of autoimmune disease after myeloablative treatment followed by autologous or syngeneic SC rescue. In particular, models of adjuvant arthritis and experimental allergic encephalomyelitis have been effectively cured after TBI followed by SCT [40, 41]. Additional evidence supporting the use of SCT as a primary therapy for autoimmune disease comes from patients where SCT was performed for haematological malignancy in the presence of a coincidental autoimmune disease.

Allogeneic SCT in patients with coincidental autoimmune disease

The beneficial response in autoimmune disease after allogeneic SCT may either be an effect of the intensive immunosuppression given as conditioning therapy or the effects of allogeneic immune reconstitution where the graft plays a role in suppression of abnormal host immune populations. Observations of patients with autoimmune disease who received unpurged allogeneic SC grafts showed that long-term remission is possible [42], though several patients eventually relapsed [42, 43] suggesting that this approach was unlikely to cure all autoimmune disease. It may be that the conditioning chemotherapy is the important factor for remission induction in patients with autoimmune disease but other factors may be more important in remission maintenance following the SCT. In particular, GVHD after allogeneic transplant may contribute to prolonged remission because of either the depression of the immune system that it causes or because of the mild immunosuppressive therapy that is needed to treat it. Low intensity, non-myeloablative regimens that permit engraftment of allogeneic SCs may reduce the mortality from allogeneic transplants and then use a "graft vs. auto-immunity" effect to treat the underlying autoimmune disease (this is done using HLA matched sibling donors) [44].

However, the mortality rate associated with allografting makes this procedure unacceptable when used primarily as a treatment for autoimmune disease, despite the encouraging results seen in some cases. For this reason, clinical studies have used the safer autologous grafts for haemopoietic rescue after high dose immunoablative chemotherapy.

Autologous SCT as primary therapy for autoimmune disease

When used as primary therapy for an autoimmune disease, SCT should only be considered when the underlying condition is severe enough to have an increased risk of mortality, but needs to be carried out before irreversible organ damage has occurred. Several autoimmune diseases have been considered to be appropriate for therapy with SCT (Tab. 2). In this broad group of diseases the theoretically most efficient approach to therapy is to use stronger myeloablation and greater T-cell depletion from the graft. However, this approach is associated with a higher mortality from ensuing immunodeficiency and a careful balance therefore exists between the clinical benefits and potential toxicity. By March 1999 there were 150 patients on the register for patients with autoimmune disease receiving a SCT. Most had received an autologous SCT (62 rheumatic disease, 47 neurological disease, eight haematological), with a response in 66% of patients and progressive disease in 22%. The treatment related death rate was 8% at 2 years [44], higher than that seen generally for other indications.

The key issues surrounding autologous PBSCT in RA were illustrated by a recent series of papers where a total of 16 patients were treated [15, 45, 46]. Each of the three groups used a slightly different approach to (a) SC mobilisation, (b) SC purification and (c) conditioning treatment prior to PBSC reinfusion. In the first study, a dramatic improvement in disease activity was seen after SC mobilisation with 4 g/m^2

Table 2 - Conditions considered suitable for stem cell transplantation

Rheumatic diseases	Neurological disease	Haematological disease
Systemic sclerosis	Myasthenia gravis	Autoimmune thrombocytopenia
Rheumatoid arthritis	Multiple sclerosis	Autoimmune haemolytic anaemia
SLE		Autoimmune neutropenia
Systemic vasculitis		Aplastic anaemia
Antiphospholipid syndrome		
Cryoglobulinaemia		
Juvenile idiopathic arthritis		

Cy alone, but partial disease relapse occurred in all patients, reaching a peak at 4–6 months [15]. This group did not proceed to SCT. A comparison of 100 mg/kg and 200 mg/kg Cy as conditioning therapy, with reinfusion of unpurged PBSC grafts, led to relapse in all patients treated with the lower Cy dose by 3–4 months [45]. Patients treated with 200 mg/kg Cy had a better and longer response, though recurrence of disease activity still occurred, suggesting that graft purging is not the only factor in relapse. Where T-cell depleted PBSC were reinfused into four patients after conditioning with Cy (200 mg/kg) and ATG (90 mg/kg), a sustained response was seen in two but disease recurred in the other two at 6 and 9 months [46].

There are important differences in the approaches used in these studies, but the overall results suggest that cure in RA is unlikely to be achieved by these approaches. This does not mean that when optimised, PBSCT does not have the potential to induce either a prolonged remission in RA or a cure in other autoimmune disease where the immunopathogenetic mechanisms are likely to differ. Importantly, rheumatoid synovitis, unlike SNV, is a particularly persistent form of autoimmune inflammation with very rare remissions, so that lessons from one disease will not necessarily apply to another.

Others have used high-dose immunosuppressive therapy (200 mg/kg Cy over 4 days) without SCT for the treatment of autoimmune disease (e.g. systemic lupus erythematosus (SLE), aplastic anaemia, pemphigoid) and have induced complete remission in their patients [16, 47, 48]. They found that haemopoietic recovery was similar to that seen after autologous PBSCT and hypothesised that the risks of disease relapse were reduced by not infusing a SC graft that may have contained auto-reactive T cells. Others have added ATG (90 mg/kg) to their conditioning Cy (200 mg/kg) and followed this up with a CD34+ve selected PBSCT for patients with refractory SLE. A total of seven patients have been treated in this way and all have achieved remissions of >1 year duration [49, 50]. The more favourable rate of remission induction in these SLE studies compared to those where the conditioning therapy was with Cy alone without SC rescue [17] may reflect the additional use of

ATG as conditioning therapy. Long-term follow-up will show what the risk of relapse is with the two approaches.

Thus, multi-centre trials with a well defined patient population and a standardised protocol acceptable to all participating units would be one approach if clear answers as to the utility of this therapy in autoimmune disease are to be obtained. However the large scale randomised controlled trial is not the ideal tool for uncommon diseases or therapies.

Why may relapse occur in autoimmune disease?

There are many possible explanations why an autoimmune disease may relapse after a SCT (Tab. 3). Persistence of autoreactive T cells in the host despite high-dose chemotherapy may precipitate relapse, as may the local persistence of other cell lines, such as monocyte/macrophages in the local (synovial) environment in RA. The latter act as antigen presenting cells, capable of immediately re-triggering an immune response unless the inflammation and associated auto-antigens can be completely cleared before immune reconstitution. If persistence of host autoreactive T cells is the mechanism for relapse then longer remissions may be induced by more aggressive conditioning immediately prior to the SCT. Alternatively, post transplant immunosuppression may also be necessary. In recipients of allogeneic grafts where there has been a degree of GVHD, a "graft vs. autoimmunity reaction" may cause ongoing inhibition of the host autoimmune reactivity thereby prolonging remission.

Relapse may also occur because of re-infusion of autoreactive T cells with the SC graft. However, there is no evidence for adoptive transfer of autoimmune disease when allogeneic BM transplants were given from patients with RA or SLE [51, 52]. Regeneration of the immune system leading to relapse of autoimmune disease (psoriasis) has been seen in a patient with a previous thymectomy, suggesting that transplantation of T cells with the graft was a possible mechanism for relapse [53]. Clinical responses may therefore be improved by post transplant immunomodulation to destroy low level residual disease and maintain remission. On the other hand an alternative, more sophisticated view of clinical auto-immunity is as a balance between "disease inducing" aberrant immune responses provoked by exogenous antigens and "disease suppressing" peripheral tolerance mechanisms. The "graft *versus* autoimmune disease" effect after allografts may be seen as an enhancement of such peripheral effects. Thus the effect of continued immunosuppressant therapy on this aspect needs elucidation, if selective immune-stimulation is really the aim.

Inherent defects in central or peripheral tolerance in the host may also be relevant as may the SC themselves if they provide intrinsic susceptibility to the autoimmune disease. As HLA type is involved in susceptibility to autoimmune disease, re-exposure to an exogenous or endogenous antigenic trigger could result in re-emer-

Table 3 - Possible reasons for relapse of autoimmune disease

Re-population by host auto-aggressive T cells
Re-population by other cell lines in host
Re-infusion of auto-aggressive T cells with SCT
Inherent susceptibility to autoimmune disease in stem cells
Re-exposure to antigenic stimulus

gence of auto-reactivity in a susceptible immune system. Thus if the putative antigenic trigger and/or defective host factors persist then relapse is inevitable, even after effective myeloablation and graft manipulation.

Stem cell transplantation in systemic vasculitis

The clinical experience of SCT in patients with SNV is limited, but additional indirect information is available from patients with RA who had associated vasculitis at the time of their SCT, probably reflecting the difference in microenvironment of synovium and blood vessel wall [15]. We believe that the questions surrounding the methodological approach used for SCT in SNV are the same as those raised for autoimmune disease in general. We must first ask why we would consider SNV patients for this aggressive, expensive approach to therapy? In some ways this can be seen as the ideal set of autoimmune diseases in which to try SCT. These are potentially lethal diseases, yet can respond well to therapy. This indicates that they are not as intrinsically persistent as the synovitis of RA. The local inflammation can be more completely suppressed and thus can be expected to go into prolonged remissions with more aggressive therapy. However, SNV has profound effects on morbidity and patient quality of life which we must aim to improve as well as survival.

Patient selection for autologous SC transplantation

It is also important to consider which patients with SNV may be suitable for such an aggressive approach to therapy. SNV are characteristically relapsing conditions, but fewer items of damage accumulate for each subsequent flare of activity, perhaps reflecting earlier presentation and institution of appropriate therapy after relapse [11]. We have turned to carefully structured high dose pulse Cy treatment with the aim of achieving a more rapid remission induction and therefore reduction of early disease related morbidity [54]. Most studies with standard Cy protocols induce remission, but the rate at which this is induced is variable with relapse still a major problem for some sub groups of SNV. However, recent European collaborative studies have shown that once remission is achieved in ANCA-associated vasculitis, azathioprine is as good as continuous oral Cy at maintaining it, without the long-term problems of drug toxicity [55]. In those SNV patients where remission can be successfully induced with short courses of Cy and maintained with milder consolidation therapy, then the costs and risks associated with high-dose immunosuppression followed by SCT would be unacceptable. Early recognition of disease activity and institution of appropriate therapy will help reduce the long-term morbidity that is still seen in this group.

Patients who have disease activity that is either unresponsive to standard Cy regimes or where frequent relapse occurs may be considered for SCT if other therapeutic avenues have been pursued. Intensification of Cy induction therapy, followed by suitable consolidation therapy, may be an effective first line option in those patients with persistent disease activity. Maintenance therapy can be improved to reduce rates of relapse by optimum use of methotrexate, azathioprine or cyclosporin (alone or in combination) and successful eradication of nasal *Staphylococcus aureus* in WG patients [56]. Those patients that fail appropriate modifications of their therapy may be suitable for autologous PBSCT if it is considered that they have life-threatening active disease that has not yet resulted in significant irreversible organ damage (e.g. renal failure). A BVAS score at first presentation of >20 has been shown to be predictive of patients with a poor prognosis [14], perhaps identifying a group where a more aggressive approach to therapy is indicated. However, these patients are also more likely to have multiple critical organ impairment, adding to the risks of the procedure. Unfortunately there is no reliable way to identify SNV patients who are going to have relapsing disease, though the incidence of relapse does appear to be disease specific. Flares of disease activity are rare in classical polyarteritis nodosa [57, 58] and some data suggests that within the ANCA-associated group of vasculitidies microscopic polyangiitis is less likely to relapse than WG. This latter disease therefore seems the most likely to be considered for SCT for relapsing disease.

Approach to stem cell transplantation in vasculitis

In general, SCT for an autoimmune disease should not be performed until consultation by two independent experts in the field has taken place and the protocol has been approved by a research ethics committee [21]. The high dose Cy doses that are used for SC mobilisation (4 g/m^2) may in fact be sufficient to induce remission without the need for conditioning chemotherapy and SC rescue, but experience with our cases suggests that this cannot be maintained without further treatment, at least in some cases. An expectant approach to treatment could be taken with SC harvesting and cryopreservation of purged CD34$^+$ cells for later use if further relapse or progression of disease occurs. Under these circumstances appropriate conditioning therapy could be used followed by SC rescue. However, the delay between harvesting and conditioning may reduce the likelihood of success of a PBSCT as the additive therapeutic effect on the local inflammatory microenvironment of the Cy used for mobilisation will be lost. Our experience with high-dose pulse therapy for remission induction shows that it is highly likely that the patient will have inactive disease when conditioning therapy is given. This clinical state is desirable as the risks of the procedure will be reduced as vital organ function will be stable. Conditioning with high-dose Cy and ATG would seem to provide the best theoretical chance of deleting all auto-reactive T cells, and in the presence of a T-cell purged graft, to provide the best chance of a cure. This approach is supported by the recent reports of ASCT in SLE where similar conditioning therapy was given with good 1 year results [49, 50].

If an autologous PBSCT, with graft purging and intensive conditioning, is performed for a patient with SNV then maintenance therapy is probably best avoided. Post-transplant immunosuppressive therapy will not only add to the risks of long-term drug toxicity but may paradoxically increase the risk of relapse. If high-dose conditioning therapy has actually achieved selective immunosuppression of the aberrant disease inducing immune function, and relative promotion of disease suppressing immune function, then post transplant immunosuppression may in fact increase the risk of relapse. In addition, strict attention should be paid to eradication of *S. aureus* from all bodily sites, perhaps reducing the risk of relapse [56].

Current experience of stem cell transplantation in vasculitis

We have personal experience of autologous PBSCT in two patients with WG, and the literature contains a small number of other case reports [20, 59]. In both Wegener's cases, recurrent relapsing disease over a number of years had lead to the accumulation of several items of organ damage. At the time of relapse in one patient there was evidence of skin, joint, sinus, lung and renal disease with both active disease and chronic scarring seen on renal biopsy. This flare was brought under rapid control by high-dose Cy but early relapse occurred and, as the patient had previously received high cumulative doses of Cy, SCT was considered. This approach was supported by the patient, his family and two independent experts and he proceeded to SC mobilisation. Two separate boluses of 5 g of Cy followed by G-CSF were necessary to achieve adequate collection of CD34$^+$ cells which were purified on a CD34$^+$ column to leave $< 0.7 \times 10^4$ CD3$^+$ cells/kg. His previous chemotherapy may have been the explanation for this poor mobilisation. Further flares in activity did not occur prior to his conditioning therapy 1 month later which was with Cy (100 mg/kg over 2 days) and Busulphan (16 mg/kg over 4 days). Two years after his transplant with 1.4×10^6 CD34$^+$ cells/kg he is still in complete clinical remission on no therapy. However he maintains cANCA positive, at a titre of 1:100 and is PR3 positive with a titre of 121 EU/ml (normal < 10). Although he had taken up full-time employment, his post transplant course has been complicated by persistent thrombocytopenia (platelets ~60 × 10^9/l), an episode of haemorrhagic cystitis which is under regular urological follow-up and avascular necrosis of his hip, presumably secondary to his previous high dose steroid therapy. The other, older WG patient was in remission for 2 years following his transplant. This was associated with a marked improvement in his quality of life as shown by a return first to sporting activities and then to work. His PB SC collection was not manipulated *in vitro* but he did receive ATG to purge the graft of T cells. Despite this approach he has recently relapsed requiring further standard dose pulse Cy.

Despite induction of a prolonged remission in the first patient, his ANCA titre has remained positive. PR3 specific ANCA has been proposed as the key putative auto-antibody in WG and its persistence has been associated with disease relapse. In contrast, lupus patients who have received successful ASCT have had a dramatic reduction in titres of auto-antibodies. This suggests that in WG, ANCA are either not the sole initiators of disease flares or that disease suppressing peripheral tolerance mechanisms, rather than central tolerance, has been enhanced by the procedure.

Other reports of high-dose immunosuppression in vasculitis include one patient with autoimmune mixed cryoglobulinaemic vasculitis with renal involvement who was treated with myeloablative doses of immunosuppressives (Cy 200 mg for 8 days + azathioprine 100 mg + prednisolone 30 mg) [20]. Pancytopenia developed by 9 days with immune regeneration by 21 days without the need for a SCT. Maintenance treatment with low dose azathioprine and cyclophosphamide was necessary to maintain remission. Allogeneic SC from a sibling were used as rescue therapy in a patient with microscopic polyangitiis after high dose chemotherapy. Remission was successfully induced but the patient was dialysis dependent because of renal damage [59].

Summary

On one hand, patients with SNV would appear to be the ideal candidates for PBSCT as lasting remissions can be induced. This is in contrast to other autoimmune diseases such as RA and SLE where lasting remissions are rarely achieved. However, with earlier diagnosis and institution of appropriate therapy, many vasculitic patients may be successfully controlled without the need for a higher risk approach. It must be remembered, however, that SNV is still associated with appreciable long-term mortality and morbidity with reduced quality of life. High-dose immunosuppression followed by SCT has the potential to provide a cure in SNV, given the right combination of graft enrichment and conditioning therapy, but this needs to be carefully balanced against the risks of transplant related morbidity and mortality. Identification of the group of individuals at highest risk of recurrent flares in activity, where accumulation of organ damage is inevitable, would allow selection of those most at risk of a poor outcome for consideration for SCT.

References

1   Breedveld FC, Daha MR (1996) Vasculitis: mechanisms of injury, In: BM Ansell, PA Bacon, JT Lie, H Yazici (eds): *The vasculitidies: science and practice*. Chapman and Hall, London, 39–47

2   Sundy JS, Haynes BF (1995) Pathogenic mechanisms of vessel damage in vasculitis syndromes. *Rheum Dis Clin North Am* 21 (4): 861–881

3   Weyand CM, Goronzy JJ (1995) Giant cell arteritis as an antigen driven disease. *Rheum Dis Clin North Am* 21: 1027–1039

4   Kallenberg CGM, Tervaert JWC, Van derWoude FJ, Goldschmeding R, Vondemborne AEGK, Weening JJ (1991) Autoimmunity to lysosomal-enzymes – new clues to vasculitis and glomerulonephritis. *Immunol Today* 12: 61–64

5   Ludviksson BR, Sneller MC, Chua KS, Talar Williams C, Langford CA, Ehrhardt RO, Fauci AS, Strober W (1998) Active Wegener's granulomatosis is associated with HLA-DR+ CD4(+) T cells exhibiting an unbalanced Th1-type T cell cytokine pattern: reversal with IL-10. *J Immunol* 160: 3602–3609

6   Lieb ES, Restivo C, Paulus HE (1979) Immunosuppressive and corticosteroid therapy of polyarteritis nodosa. *Am J Med* 67: 941–947

7   Fauci AS, Katz P, Haynes BF, Wolff SM (1979) Cyclophosphamide therapy of severe systemic necrotising vasculitis. *N Engl J Med* 301: 235–238

8   Hoffman GS, Kerr GS, Leavitt RY, Hallahan CW, Lebovics RS, Travis WD, Rottem M, Fauci AS (1992) Wegener granulomatosis – an analysis of 158 patients. *Ann Intern Med* 116: 488–498

9   Talar-Williams C, Hijazi YM, Walther MM, Linehan WM, Hallahan CW, Lubensky I, Kerr GS, Hoffman GS, Fauci AS, Sneller MC (1996) Cyclophosphamide-induced cystitis and bladder cancer in patients with Wegener granulomatosis. *Ann Intern Med* 124: 477–484

10 Adu D, Pall A, Luqmani RA, Richards NT, Howie AJ, Emery P, Michael J, Savage CO, Bacon PA (1997) Controlled trial of pulse versus continuous prednisolone and cyclophosphamide in the treatment of systemic vasculitis. *QJM* 90: 401–409

11 Exley AR, Carruthers DM, Luqmani RA, Kitas GD, Gordon C, Janssen BA, Savage COS, Bacon PA (1997) Damage occurs early in systemic vasculitis and is an index of outcome. *QJM* 90: 391–399

12 Mullins GM, Colvin M (1975) Intensive cyclophosphamide (NSC-26271) therapy for solid tumours. *Cancer Chemotherapy Reports* 59: 411–419

13 Hoffman GS (1993) Wegener's granulomatosis. *Curr Opin Rheumatol* 5: 11–17

14 Luqmani RA, Bacon PA, Moots RJ, Janssen BA, Pall A, Emery P, Savage C, Adu D (1994) Birmingham Vasculitis Activity Score (BVAS) in systemic necrotizing vasculitis. *QJM* 87: 671–678

15 Breban M, Dougados M, Picard F, Marolleau JP, Bocaccio C, Heshmati F, Dreyfus F, Bouscary D (1999) Intensified dose cyclophosphamide (id-hdc) and G-CSF administration for hematopoietic stem cell (HSC) mobilization in refractory rheumatoid arthritis (RA). *Arthritis Rheum* 42: 992

16 Brodsky RA, Sensenbrenner LL, Jones RJ (1996) Complete remission in severe aplastic anemia after high-dose cyclophosphamide without bone marrow transplantation. *Blood* 87: 491–494

17 Petri M, Jones A, Brodsky R (1999) High-dose immunoablative cyclophosphamide in SLE. *Arthritis Rheum* 42: S170 (Abstract)

18 Brouwer E, Huitema MG, Mulder AHL, Heeringa P, Vangoor H, Tervaert JWC, Weening JJ, Kallenberg CGM (1994) Neutrophil activation *in vitro* and *in vivo* in Wegener's granulomatosis. *Kidney Internat* 45: 1120–1131

19 Kovarsky J (1983) Clinical pharmacology and toxicology of cyclophosphamide – emphasis on use in rheumatic diseases. *Semin Arthritis Rheum* 12: 359–372

20 Slavin S (1993) Treatment of life-threatening autoimmune-diseases with myeloablative doses of immunosuppressive agents – experimental background and rationale for ABMT. *Bone Marrow Transplant* 12: 85–88

21 Tyndall A, Gratwohl A (1997) Blood and marrow stem cell transplants in autoimmune disease – a consensus report written on behalf of the European league against rheumatism (EULAR) and the European group for blood and marrow transplantation (EBMT). *Br J Rheumatol* 36: 390–392

22 Majolino I, Pearce R, Taghipour G, Goldstone AH (1997) Peripheral blood stem cell transplantation versus autologous bone marrow transplantation in Hodgkin's and non-Hodgkin's lymphomas: a new matched pair analysis of the European group for blood and marrow transplantation registry data. *J Clin Oncol* 15: 509–517

23 Platzer E (1989) Human haematopoietic growth factors. *Eur J Haematol* 42: 1–15

24 Gianni AM, Bregni M, Siena S, Villa S, Sciorelli GA, Ravagnani F, Pellegris G, Bonadonna G (1989) Rapid and complete hematopoietic reconstitution following combined transplantation of autologous blood and bone-marrow cells – a changing-role for high-dose chemo-radiotherapy. *Hematol Oncology* 7: 139–148

25 Cantin G, Marchandlaroche D, Bouchard MM, Leblond PF (1989) Blood-derived stem-cell collection in acute non lymphoblastic leukemia – predictive factors for a good yield. *Exp Hematol* 17: 991–996

26 Snowden JA, Biggs JC, Milliken ST, Fuller A, Staniforth D, Passuello F, Renwick J, Brooks PM (1998) A randomised, blinded, placebo-controlled, dose escalation study of the tolerability and efficacy of filgrastim for haemopoietic stem cell mobilisation in patients with severe active rheumatoid arthritis. *Bone Marrow Transplant* 22: 1035–1041

27 Kernan NA, Collins NH, Juliano L, Cartagena T, Dupont B, Oreilly RJ (1986) Clonable lymphocytes in T-cell-depleted bone-marrow transplants correlate with development of graft-v-host disease. *Blood* 68: 770–773

28 Kardamakis D, Berry RJ (1987) Low-dose total-body irradiation in rheumatoid-arthritis. *Br J Rheumatol* 26: 234–235

29 Roux E, Helg C, Dumont Girard F, Chapuis B, Jeannet M, Roosnek E (1996) Analysis of T-cell repopulation after allogeneic bone marrow transplantation: significant differences between recipients of T-cell depleted and unmanipulated grafts. *Blood* 87: 3984–3992

30 Mackall CL, Fleisher TA, Brown MR, Andrich MP, Chen CC, Feuerstein IM, Horowitz ME, Magrath IT, Shad AT, Steinberg SM et al (1995) Age, thymopoiesis, and CD4$^+$ T-lymphocyte regeneration after intensive chemotherapy. *N Engl J Med* 332: 143–149

31 Collins RH (1997) Autologous haemopoietic stem cell transplantation. *Lancet* 349: 881

32 Mackall CL, Hakim FT, Gress RE (1997) T-cell regeneration: all repertoires are not created equal. *Immunol Today* 18: 245–251

33 Miller RA, Stutman O (1984) T-cell repopulation from functionally restricted splenic progenitors – 10,000-fold expansion documented by using limiting dilution analyses. *J Immunol* 133: 2925–2932

34 Bomberger C, Singh Jairam M, Rodey G, Guerriero A, Yeager AM, Fleming WH, Holland HK, Waller EK (1998) Lymphoid reconstitution after autologous PBSC transplantation with facs-sorted CD34(+) hematopoietic progenitors. *Blood* 91: 2588–2600

35 Gorski J, Yassai M, Zhu XL, Kissella B, Keever C, Flomenberg N (1994) Circulating T-cell repertoire complexity in normal individuals and bone-marrow recipients analyzed by CDR3 size spectra typing – correlation with immune status. *J Immunol* 152: 5109–5119

36 Forman SJ, Nocker P, Gallagher M, Zaia J, Wright C, Bolen J, Mills B, Hecht T (1982) Pattern of T-cell reconstitution following allogeneic bone-marrow transplantation for acute hematological malignancy. *Transplant* 34: 96–98

37 Anderson KC, Soiffer R, Delage R, Takvorian T, Freedman AS, Rabinowe SL, Nadler LM, Dear K, Heflin L, Mauch P et al (1990) T-cell-depleted autologous bone-marrow transplantation therapy – analysis of immune-deficiency and late complications. *Blood* 76: 235–244

38 Keever CA, Small TN, Flomenberg N, Heller G, Pekle K, Black P, Pecora A, Gillio A, Kernan NA, Oreilly RJ (1989) Immune reconstitution following bone-marrow transplantation – comparison of recipients of T-cell depleted marrow with recipients of conventional marrow grafts. *Blood* 73: 1340–1350

39 Olsen GA, Gockerman JP, Bast RC, Borowitz M, Peters WP (1988) Altered immunological reconstitution after standard-dose chemotherapy or high-dose chemotherapy with autologous bone-marrow support. *Transplantation* 46: 57–60

40 Van Bekkum DW, Bohre EPM, Houben PFJ, Knaanshanzer S (1989) Regression of adjuvant-induced arthritis in rats following bone-marrow transplantation. *PNAS* 86: 10090–10094

41 Van Gelder M, Kinwelbohre EPM, Van Bekkum DW (1993) Treatment of experimental allergic encephalomyelitis in rats with total-body irradiation and syngeneic BMT. *Bone Marrow Transplant* 11: 233–241

42 Snowden JA, Kearney P, Kearney A, Cooley HM, Grigg A, Jacobs P, Bergman J, Brooks PM, Biggs JC (1998) Long-term outcome of autoimmune disease following allogeneic bone marrow transplantation. *Arthritis Rheum* 41: 453–459

43 Cooley HM, Snowden JA, Grigg AP, Wicks IP (1997) Outcome of rheumatoid arthritis and psoriasis following autologous stem cell transplantation for hematologic malignancy. *Arthritis Rheum* 40: 1712–1715

44 Snowden JA, Brooks PM (1999) Hematopoietic stem cell transplantation in rheumatic diseases. *Curr Opin Rheumatol* 11: 167–172

45 Snowden JA, Biggs JC, Milliken ST, Fuller A, Brooks PM (1999) A phase I/II dose escalation study of intensified cyclophosphamide and autologous blood stem cell rescue in severe, active rheumatoid arthritis. *Arthritis Rheum* 42: 2286–2292

46 Burt RK, Georganas C, Schroeder J, Traynor A, Stefka J, Schuening F, Graziano F, Mineishi S, Cheng D, Rosen S et al (1999) Autologous hematopoietic stem cell transplantation of refractory rheumatoid arthritis. *Arthritis Rheum* 42: 33

47 Brodsky RA, Petri M, Smith BD, Seifter EJ, Spivak JL, Styler M, Dang CV, Brodsky I, Jones RJ (1998) Immunoablative high-dose cyclophosphamide without stem-cell rescue for refractory, severe autoimmune disease. *Ann Intern Med* 129: 1031–1035

48 Nousari HC, Brodsky RA, Jones RJ, Grever MR, Anhalt GJ (1999) Immunoablative high-dose cyclophosphamide without stem cell rescue in paraneoplastic pemphigus: report of a case and review of this new therapy for severe autoimmune disease. *J Am Acad Dermatol* 40: 750–754

49 Hiepe F, Rosen O, Thiel A, Massenkeil G, Radtke H, Haupl T, Gromnica-Ihle E, Radbruch A, Arnold R (1999) Successful treatment of refractory systemic lupus erythematosus (SLE) by autologous stem cell transplantation (ASCT) with *in vivo* immunomodulation and *ex vivo* depletion of mononuclear cells. *Arthritis Rheum* 42: S170 (Abstract)

50 Traynor AE, Schroder J, Rosa RM, Mujais S, Rosen S, Bowyer S, Jung L, Burt R (1999) Stem cell transplantation for resistant lupus. *Arthritis Rheum* 42: S170 (Abstract)

51 Snowden JA, Atkinson K, Kearney P, Brooks P, Briggs JC (1997) Allogeneic bone marrow transplantation from a donor with severe active rheumatoid arthritis not resulting in adoptive transfer of disease to recipient. *Bone Marrow Transplant* 20: 71–73

52 Sturfelt G, Lenhoff S, Sallerfors B, Nived O, Truedsson L, Sjoholm AG (1996) Transplantation with allogenic bone marrow from a donor with systemic lupus erythematosus (SLE): successful outcome in the recipient and induction of an SLE flare in the donor. *Ann Rheum Dis* 55: 638–641

53 Euler HH, Marmont AM, Bacigalupo A, Fastenrath S, Dreger P, Hoffknecht M, Zander AR, Schalke B, Hahn U, Haas R et al (1996) Early recurrence or persistence of autoimmune diseases after unmanipulated autologous stem cell transplantation. *Blood* 88: 3621–3625

54 Carruthers DM, Exley AR, Williams R, Buckley CD, Amft N, Raza K, Rowe I, Bacon PA (1998) Intensive pulse cyclophosphamide for remission induction in systemic necrotising vasculitis (SNV). *Arthritis Rheum* 41: 545 (Abstract)

55 Luqmani R, Jayne D (1999) A multi-centre randomised trial of cyclophosphamide versus azathioprine during remission in anca-associated systemic vasculitis (cycazarem). *Arthritis Rheum* 42: 928 (Abstract)

56 Stegeman CA, Tervaert JWC, de Jong PE, Kallenberg CGM (1996) Trimethoprim-sulfamethoxazole (co-trimoxazole) for the prevention of relapses of Wegener's granulomatosis. *N Engl J Med* 335: 16–20

57 Gayraud M, Guillevin L, Cohen P, Lhote F, Cacoub P, Deblois P, Godeau B, Ruel M, Vidal E, Piontud M et al (1997) Treatment of good-prognosis polyarteritis nodosa and Churg-Strauss syndrome: comparison of steroids and oral or pulse cyclophosphamide in 25 patients. French Cooperative Study Group for Vasculitides. *Br J Rheumatol* 36: 1290–1297

58 Guillevin L, Lhote F, Cohen P, Jarrousse B, Lortholary O, Genereau T, Leon A, Bussel A (1995) Corticosteroids plus pulse cyclophosphamide and plasma exchanges versus corticosteroids plus pulse cyclophosphamide alone in the treatment of polyarteritis nodosa and Churg-Strauss syndrome patients with factors predicting poor prognosis. A prospective, randomized trial in sixty-two patients. *Arthritis Rheum* 38: 1638–1645

59 Fastenrath S, Schroder JO, Uharek L, Dreger P, Glass B, Harten P, Schmitz N, Euler HH (1997) Transplantation of allogeneic stem cells in a patient with severe microscopic polyarteritis. *Arthritis Rheum* 40: 815 (Abstract)

Prevention of relapsing disease in anti-neutrophil cytoplasmic antibody related necrotizing small-vessel vasculitis: the role for autoantibody guided and anti-bacterial treatment

Maarten M. Boomsma[1], Coen A. Stegeman[2], Cees G.M. Kallenberg[1] and Jan W. Cohen Tervaert[3]

Department of Internal Medicine, [1]Division of Clinical Immunology, [2]Division of Nephrology, University Hospital Groningen, 9713 GZ Groningen, The Netherlands; [3]Department of Internal Medicine, Division of Clinical Immunology, University Hospital Maastricht, 6202 AZ Maastricht, The Netherlands

Introduction

Within the spectrum of primary vasculitic syndromes, the anti-neutrophil cytoplasmic antibody (ANCA) related syndromes form a distinct group with overlapping features. ANCA related small-vessel vasculitides are potentially life-threatening diseases with high mortality. Prolonged immunosuppressive therapy (> 1 year) with cyclophosphamide and steroids is effective in inducing disease remission and preventing early relapses in most vasculitic disorders [1–6]. Continuous use of cyclophosphamide to sustain remission cannot be recommended, however, since this treatment regimen is associated with severe and potentially lethal adverse effects such as the occurrence of opportunistic infections and the development of malignancies [7, 8]. Therefore, cyclophosphamide is tapered or stopped once remission is achieved to prevent adverse effects. Alternatively, azathioprine may be used as maintenance therapy after a remission is induced with cyclophosphamide and steroids [5]. Azathioprine is considered less effective in inducing remission than cyclophosphamide, but its long-term toxicity is much lower [9, 10]. The potential of azathioprine as maintenance therapy was recently investigated and compared with cyclophosphamide in a large randomized trial (CYCAZAREM) [11–13]. Following induction therapy with oral cyclophosphamide and steroids, maintenance treatment with azathioprine was as effective as the continued use of cyclophosphamide in the prevention of disease relapse during a 15-month follow-up period in this study. Other alternative maintenance therapy regimens, such as methotrexate [14], cyclosporin A [15], or mycophenolate [16] have been described but have not been tested adequately until now.

Since relapses may occur after azathioprine is stopped, prolonged prophylactic treatment with few adverse-effects is desirable. The potential of azathioprine as long-term maintenance therapy after remission is induced is currently investigated in a large randomized controlled trial (REMAIN) in which azathioprine is compared with a strategy in which the patients do not receive any maintenance therapy after 15 months [11].

A major disadvantage of prolonged maintenance therapy is that this therapy may expose a substantial number of patients to the unnecessary risk of drug-related morbidity. Some patients do not suffer from a relapse, whereas in patients with a relapse the interval between remission and occurrence of first relapse may vary from 3 months to 16 years [4]. A cost-benefit argument for exposure to this treatment is, on the other hand, the observation that relapses are associated with substantial morbidity and mortality [17]. Risk-adjusted treatment by successful prediction of relapses and prevention of relapses by pre-emptive therapy could be of great clinical importance. In this chapter we will review the relevant literature on this subject.

What is a relapse and what is a remission?

Vasculitides are an extraordinary heterogeneous group of inflammatory disorders with diverse clinical manifestations. The vasculitic process can affect blood vessels of any type, size or location, and therefore can cause dysfunction in virtually any organ system. Thus, scoring systems for assessing disease extent and activity are clearly wanted. The purpose of the Disease Extent Index (DEI) [18] is to assess the extent of vasculitis involvement, rather than its activity *per se*. At least three groups created indices for measurement of vasculitis activity. We proposed an activity score to measure activity in Wegener's granulomatosis [19]. Subsequently, the Birmingham Vasculitis Activity Score (BVAS) [20] and the Vasculitis Activity Index (VAI) [21] were designed to measure the level of activity in patients with all forms of active systemic necrotizing vasculitis. All three indices are valuable in assessing the extent and severity of disease, but have their limitations in defining a relapse or remission. In the literature, the definition of a relapse of vasculitis varies between studies. In many studies, no [2, 4] or only a rough description is given such as "re-emerging of clinical symptoms of vasculitis after a period of complete remission" [22–26]. In only a few studies precise and well-defined criteria for the definition of a relapse have been given [27–32].

The occurrence of relapses

In many studies data on relapses in patients with various forms of ANCA associated small-vessel vasculitis have been published [2, 4, 22–29, 31–34]. The number of patients suffering from one or more relapses during follow-up, after achieving complete remission, ranges from 25–81%. Differences in patient selection, duration of follow-up, definition of disease activity, and immunosuppressive treatment protocols may underlie the large variability in relapse rates. Hoffman et al. performed the largest observational study [4]. In this study, 158 patients with Wegener's granulomatosis were studied from diagnosis, during a follow-up of up to 24 years. Cyclophosphamide was continued for at least 1 year after the patient achieved complete remission, and then tapered every 2 to 3 months. With this treatment regimen, 66% of the patients with Wegener's granulomatosis with over 5 years of follow-up after diagnosis experienced at least one relapse, whereas more than 80% of the patients with over 10 years of follow-up experienced one or more relapses. In a recent study by Reinhold-Keller et al., 99 out of 155 (64%) patients with Wegener's granulomatosis with a median follow-up of 7 years (ranging from 0.3 to 27.3 years) suffered from one or more relapses during follow-up, 50 after complete remission, 49 after partial remission [26]. In this study, after partial or complete remission was achieved, cyclophosphamide treatment was switched to long-term maintenance regimens with co-trimoxazole in patients with normal renal function who were not taking steroids, methotrexate in patients in partial remission with restored renal function or azathioprine in patients with impaired renal function. Gordon et al. studied 150 consecutive patients with various forms of systemic vasculitis presenting over a 10-year period [22]. The follow-up ranged from 1 month up to 9.75 years. Twenty-seven patients died within 3 months of diagnosis. Of the remaining 123 patients, 42 (34%) had one or more relapses during follow-up. Gordon et al. found that the relapse risk was diagnosis dependent. Patients with limited Wegener's granulomatosis (without renal disease) and generalized Wegener's granulomatosis (with renal disease) showed a higher risk of suffering from a relapse than patients with other forms of vasculitis such as microscopic polyangiitis. The relapse rates of patients with limited Wegener's granulomatosis and generalized Wegener's granulomatosis were 52% (median time to relapse 18 months) and 44% (median time to relapse 42 months), respectively, whereas the relapse rate of patients with microscopic polyangiitis was only 25% (median time to relapse 24 months). Nachman et al. studied 97 patients with microscopic polyangiitis and idiopathic necrotizing crescentic glomerulonephritis for a mean of 2.7 years [29]. Of the 75 patients that went into remission, 22 (29%) suffered a relapse which occurred within 18 months of the end of therapy. Guillevin et al. studied 96 patients with Churg-Strauss syndrome [24]. Of their 86 patients coming into remission, 22 (26%) suffered a relapse that occurred after a mean interval from remission to relapse of 5.8 years.

Geffriaud-Ricourd et al. studied the course of the disease in 76 patients with various forms of ANCA associated vasculitis for a mean period of 2.5 years [35]. Relapses occurred in 36% of patients with Proteinase-3 (PR3)-ANCA PR3-ANCA and 20% of patients with myeloperoxidase (MPO)-ANCA. Franssen et al. studied 92 patients with ANCA associated vasculitis and in this study patients with PR3-ANCA associated vasculitis had a significantly higher relapse rate (22%) than patients with MPO-ANCA associated vasculitis (7%) (follow-up not stated) [36]. Westman et al. studied 123 patents with Wegener's granulomatosis and microscop-

Table 1 - The occurrence of relapses in patients with ANCA associated vasculitis

Reference	n.	Patients with (a) relapse(s)	Number of relapses	Follow-up (years) Median (range)	Relapses/ years
[27]	35	12 (34%)	17	1.3 (1.3)	0.26/year
[28]	57	23 (40%)	32	3.5 (1.2–3.5)	0.18/year
[32]	100	37 (37%)	48	2.9 (1.1–3.0)	0.18/year

ic polyangiitis with biopsy proven renal involvement for a mean of 5.3 years and they also found a tendency to higher relapse rates in patients with PR3-ANCA than in those with MPO-ANCA, however this was not statistically significant [31].

At our institution, several studies were published with data on relapses in patients with Wegener's granulomatosis (Tab. 1). In these studies, patients were included when remission was induced after initial diagnosis or relapse [27, 32], or inclusion occurred irrespective of disease activity [28]. Therefore, these data are not comparable with studies described above, in which patients were studied from onset of disease.

Risk factors for relapses

The literature pertaining to risk factors and preventive treatment strategies for relapses is largely restricted to patients with ANCA associated vasculitis, especially to patients with (PR3-ANCA positive) Wegener's granulomatosis. Whether findings are also applicable to patients with MPO-ANCA positive vasculitis or other forms of vasculitis remains largely unknown.

Anti neutrophil cytoplasmic antibodies (ANCA) as a risk factor for relapses

ANCA were first described in 1982 by Davies et al. in a few patients with necrotizing crescentic glomerulonephritis [37]. In 1985, van der Woude et al. showed that ANCA producing a cytoplasmic staining pattern on ethanol-fixed neutrophils using the indirect immunofluorescence technique (IIF) are a sensitive marker for Wegener's granulomatosis [38]. Subsequently, ANCA producing a perinuclear cytoplasmic staining pattern (P-ANCA) by IIF were described in patients with idiopathic necrotizing crescentic glomerulonephritis, microscopic polyangiitis, and Churg Strauss syndrome [39, 40]. PR3 and MPO were identified in these patients as the principal target antigens of C-ANCA and P-ANCA, respectively, in those diseases [39, 40].

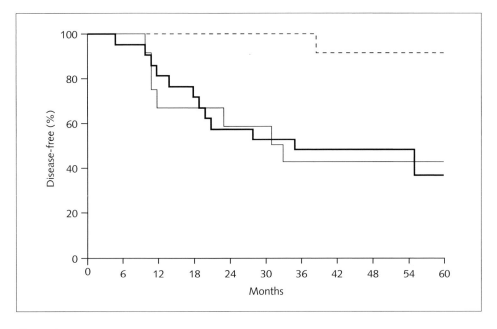

Figure 1
Disease-free interval and C-ANCA status. Disease-free interval according to the course of C-ANCA during the study (n = 54). The time of disease-free interval was counted from the beginning of the most recent period of disease activity (either initial diagnosis or relapse). (C-ANCA-negative versus *intermittently and persistently C-ANCA-positive, p < 0.001). Dashed line = C-ANCA-negative (n = 21); broad line = intermittently C-ANCA positive (n = 21); thin line = persistently C-ANCA-positive (n = 12). Reprinted from [28] with permission of the publisher.*

Although there is clinically considerable overlap, PR3-ANCA associated vasculitis predominantly relates to patients who have vasculitis that is associated with upper respiratory tract disease (Wegener's granulomatosis), whereas MPO-ANCA associated vasculitis mainly relates to patients with idiopathic necrotizing crescentic glomerulonephritis and microscopic polyangiitis with limited extrarenal organ involvement [41].

Van der Woude et al. suggested in 1985 that levels of C-ANCA as measured by IIF parallel disease activity [38]. Indeed, in patients with newly diagnosed disease high levels are observed and these levels decline during immunosuppressive treatment and become undetectable in many cases [27]. In some patients, however, ANCA levels are persistently detectable without any sign or symptom of active disease. The persistence of ANCA has been identified as a risk factor for an ensuing relapse by several groups (Fig. 1) [28, 34, 42]. Persistent positivity may also be a risk

Table 2 - Relationship between relapses and rises in ANCA as detected by indirect immunofluorescence (IIF)

Reference	n.	ANCA staining pattern (IIF)	Relapse preceded by a rise in ANCA	Rise in ANCA followed by a relapse
[27]	35	C-ANCA	100%	77%
[44]	10	C-ANCA	100%	75%
[45]	58	C-ANCA	90%	82%
[46]	10	N.R.	82%	65%
[33]	68	C-ANCA	24%	56%
[23]	37	C/P-ANCA	43%	23%
[25]	19	C-ANCA	N.R.	57%
[32]	85	C-ANCA	52%	57%

N.R., not reported; C-ANCA, cytoplasmic staining pattern; P-ANCA pattern, perinuclear
staining pattern

factor for the development of end stage renal failure in the absence of signs of a relapse of disease as was found in patients with MPO-ANCA associated necrotizing crescentic glomerulonephritis [43].

Furthermore, we noted that rises in C-ANCA titer as detected by IIF often precedes disease activity when ANCA levels are serially measured. In our first study, 17 relapses in 35 patients were observed and all (100%) were preceded by a significant rise in C-ANCA titer [27]. Furthermore, out of 22 C-ANCA rises, 17 (77%) were followed by a relapse. These early findings suggested that serial measurement of ANCA titers is useful in the follow-up of patients with Wegener's granulomatosis. After this study, several other groups have reported on the clinical utility of serial measurements of ANCA as detected by IIF (Tab. 2). Differences in frequency of ANCA testing, use of immunosuppressive maintenance therapy, and methodology of ANCA testing may underlie the large variability in results. In a pooled analysis of published data from the studies listed in Table 2 [23, 25, 27, 32, 33, 44–46], 59% of relapses were preceded by rising titers, whereas only 48% of rises in ANCA titers as measured by IIF were followed by a relapse. In our recent prospective study on a large cohort of 85 patients with C-ANCA positive Wegener's granulomatosis, 33 relapses were observed and 17 (52%) were preceded by a significant rise in C-ANCA titer (IIF). Furthermore, of the 30 significant rises in C-ANCA (IIF), 17 (57%) were followed by a relapse (Fig. 2) [32].

The IIF technique has the disadvantage that levels of ANCA are difficult to quantify precisely [33, 47]. Solid phase assays using purified antigens are better suited to quantify specific antibody levels. Four studies using serial determination of ANCA

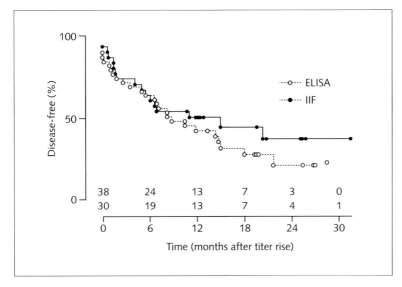

Figure 2
Percentage of patients with Wegener's granulomatosis who did not experience disease relapses in the indicated time period after a rise in antineutrophil cytoplasmic antibodies as measured by either indirect immunofluorescence (● IIF; n = 30) or antigen-specific enzyme-linked immunosorbent assay (o ELISA; n = 38). The numbers above the horizontal axis indicate the number of patients who were still at risk for a relapse at 6, 12, 18, 24, and 30 months after the rise in antibody levels as detected by ELISA (upper numbers) or IIF (lower numbers). Reprinted from [32] with permission of the publisher.

by ELISA have been published and are listed in Table 3 [25, 32, 34, 42]. Substantial differences are noted in the methodology of ANCA testing. De'Oliviera et al. [34] used an extract of azurophilic granules as antigen to measure ANCA levels, whereas in the other studies purified antigens (PR3 or MPO) were used [25, 32, 42]. Furthermore, patients with different forms of ANCA-associated vasculitis were studied, i.e., either only patients with Wegener's granulomatosis [32], patients with Wegener's granulomatosis and microscopic polyangiitis [42], patients with Wegener's granulomatosis, microscopic polyangiitis and renal limited vasculitis [25], or patients with Wegener's granulomatosis, microscopic polyangiitis, renal limited vasculitis and Churg-Strauss syndrome [34]. Jayne et al. found rises in ANCA prior to or at the moment of a relapse in 74% of the patients; in 45% of the cases those rises preceded clinical symptoms [42]. In this study, patient follow-up was restricted to the first year after diagnosis. In the study of Kyndt et al., 73% of MPO-ANCA positive patients had a rise in ANCA prior to or at the moment of relapse (in 55% of the cases rises preceded clinical symptoms), whereas only 33% of the PR3-ANCA

Table 3 - Relationship between relapses and rises in ANCA as detected enzyme linked immunosorbent assay (ELISA)

Reference	n.	ANCA specificity	Relapse preceded by a rise in ANCA	Rise in ANCA followed by a relapse
[34]	56	Extract	41%	62%
[42]	60	N.R.	74%	79%
[25]	17	PR3	33%	59%
	19	MPO	73%	79%
[32]	85	PR3	81%	71%
	15	MPO	75%	100%

N.R., not reported; PR3, proteinase 3; MPO, myeloperoxidase; extract, extract of azurophilic granules

positive patients had a rise in ANCA as detected by ELISA prior to or at the moment of relapse (preceding clinical symptoms in 20%) [25]. Unfortunately, in this latter study no precise definitions were given for ANCA rises and inter-assay variation was not reported. Furthermore, the patients were sampled with intervals as long as 3 months, which might explain why many rises in ANCA were found at the time of the relapse instead of prior to the relapse. In our study, we found that 82% of the patients with PR3-ANCA associated Wegener's granulomatosis had a rise in ANCA as detected by ELISA prior to or at the moment of a relapse (preceding clinical symptoms in 66%), and that 71% of the PR3-ANCA rises were followed by a relapse (Fig. 2) [32]. Furthermore, 75% of the relapses in patients with MPO-ANCA associated Wegener's granulomatosis were preceded by a rise in MPO-ANCA, and all MPO-ANCA rises were followed by a relapse. There is, however, great variability in time lag between the detection of a rise in ANCA and the occurrence of a relapse. In the study of Jayne et al., a rise in ANCA preceded the clinical relapse by 7.8 weeks (standard deviation 6.5 weeks) in 57% of the patients with a relapse, and in 17% of their patients ANCA rose at the time of a relapse [42]. Although, during extended follow-up, a relapse occurred in 71% of patients after a rise in PR3-ANCA (ELISA) in our prospective study, only 39% of the patients with such a rise had a relapse of their disease within 6 months after the rise, and 59% of the patients within 12 months [32]. The median time between the detection of a rise in PR3-ANCA and a relapse was 167 days (range 0–616 days) and the interval between a rise in MPO-ANCA and a relapse ranged from 121 to 217 days.

Overall, it can be concluded that relapses are frequently preceded by increases of ANCA, and that ELISA is a more sensitive method than IIF in predicting disease

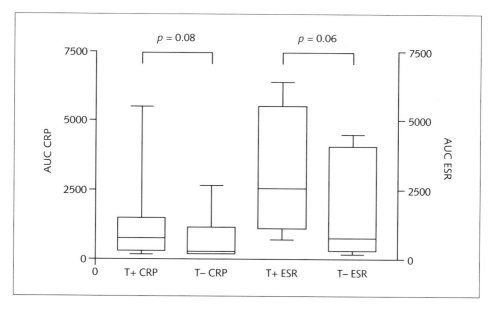

Figure 3
Area under the curve (AUC) of C-reactive protein (CRP) levels (mg/l) and erythrocyte sedi-
mentation rate (ESR) (mm/hour) during a 3-month period in patients with a rise in PR3-
ANCA (T+) not followed by a relapse of disease activity as compared to matched patients
without a rise (T–). Patients with a rise in PR3-ANCA had slightly higher C-reactive protein
levels (p = 0.08) and erythrocyte sediment rates (p = 0.06) as compared to the controls.

activity. However, ANCA increases are not invariably followed by a relapse (Tabs. 2 and 3). Why are rising ANCA titers not always followed by a relapse? It has been reported that switching from cyclophosphamide to azathioprine therapy may result in a rise in ANCA that is not followed by a relapse [42]. Another explanation could be that patients with a rise in ANCA may have subtle signs of disease activity but do not fulfill the criteria for a relapse. In our study, we observed a rise in PR3-ANCA (ELISA) that was not followed by a relapse in 11 patients [32]. These 11 patients had slightly higher C-reactive protein levels and erythrocyte sedimentation rates during the first 3 months after an ANCA rise than 11 age and sex matched patients with Wegener's granulomatosis without a rise in ANCA in the same period (Fig. 3) (unpublished data). Therefore, we hypothesize that these patients may have suffered from low-grade disease activity after an ANCA rise.

Since high ANCA levels may be found in patients during clinical remission, we postulate that differences in qualities of antibodies may be important with respect to the development of a relapse. Previously, it was found that IgG isolated from serum samples of patients with active generalized Wegener's granulomatosis, when incubated with donor granulocytes, induced significantly higher levels of the respiratory burst compared with IgG isolated from patients in remission [48]. Changes in the capacity to induce the respiratory burst were not related to ANCA levels as measured by IIF and/or ELISA, but were related to the IgG3 ANCA/total IgG ANCA ratio. Furthermore we demonstrated in a small retrospective study that rises in IgG3 subclass of ANCA as measured by ELISA were a more specific predictor of relapses than rises of C-ANCA as measured by IIF [49]. However, in our recent large prospective study we found that additional measurement of levels of IgG3 subclass of PR3-ANCA was of little benefit [32]. Rises in levels of IgG3 subclass of PR3-ANCA increased the positive predictive value of a rise in ANCA, but decreased the sensitivity for a relapse. Anti-PR3 antibodies interfere with the complexation of PR3 with α-1 antitrypsin [50]. In a longitudinal study it was shown that disease activity in patients with Wegener's granulomatosis correlates with the capacity of the antibodies to inhibit complexation rather than with the titer of the anti-PR3 antibodies as detected by either IIF or ELISA [51]. Anti-PR3 antibodies also interfere with PR3 elastinolytic and proteolytic activity [50]. Inhibitory activity of the antibodies changes during the course of the disease, reflecting disease activity better than the absolute anti-PR3 titer [52]. All these studies support the idea that not only the quantity, but also the quality of ANCA might influence the pathogenic potential of the antibodies.

Infections as a risk factor for relapses

Patients with Wegener's granulomatosis frequently have symptoms of respiratory tract infections at the time of an ANCA rise [45], at the onset of the disease, or preceding the occurrence of a relapse [37, 53, 54]. So, does infection trigger relapses in Wegener's granulomatosis? Previously, we found that nine out of 23 patients with a relapse had an upper-airway infection during a 6 months period preceding the relapse. However, infections were not specifically associated with relapses since many infections were not related to a relapse [28]. This was also found in another longitudinal study of 81 patients with Wegener's granulomatosis [30]. We conclude from these studies that infections are not important triggers for relapses although it is possible that self-limiting viral or bacterial infections have been missed in patients.

However, virtually every patient with Wegener's granulomatosis has a low-grade chronic infection of the nasal mucosa, predominantly caused by *Staphylococcus aureus* (*S. aureus*). Our group demonstrated that there is an association between chronic nasal carriage of *S. aureus* and an increased frequency of relapses during follow-up (Fig. 4) [28]. Others also found an association between nasal carriage of *S. aureus* and activity of Wegener's granulomatosis in the upper respiratory tract [55].

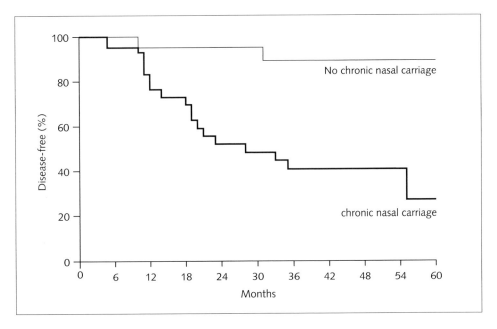

Figure 4
Disease-free interval and carrier status. Disease-free interval of 57 patients with Wegener's granulomatosis grouped according to Staphylococcus aureus carrier status. The time of disease free-interval was counted from the beginning of the most recent period of disease activity (either initial diagnosis or relapse; p < 0.001). Reprinted from [28] with permission of the publisher.

Other possible risk factors

Various other risk factors have been identified. Previous studies have produced conflicting findings about the association between renal function and relapses in patients with Wegener's granulomatosis. Previously we found that a creatinine clearance above 60 ml/min is an independent risk factor for relapse [28]. We could not confirm this finding in our recent study [32] and, on the other hand, Hogan et al. found that a high serum creatinine level at the end of therapy is associated with a higher risk of relapse [56]. Thus, the relation between renal function and risk factors for relapses is presently not clear. Another risk factor relates to functional polymorphism in receptors for the Fc-fragment of IgG (Fcγ receptor). Analysis of polymorphisms in phenotype of Fcγ receptors demonstrated that patients with Wegener's granulomatosis were more prone to disease relapse in the first 5 years after diagnosis if they were homozygous for both the R131 form of Fcγ receptor IIa and the F158 form of Fcγ receptor IIIa (relative risk 3.3, 95% confidence interval 1.6–

6.8) [57]. These polymorphisms are both associated with decreased Fc-receptor-mediated clearance, which may be relevant to the persistence of nasal carriage of *S. aureus*. Finally, Hogan et al. also identified upper respiratory tract involvement in small-vessel vasculitis as a risk factor for the development of relapses [56].

Prevention of relapses

Antibody directed treatment

Since many patients with a rise in ANCA will suffer from a relapse, one may question whether treatment based on changes in ANCA levels might be justified. In 1990, we reported that treatment with steroids and cyclophosphamide based on rises in C-ANCA (IIF) could prevent the occurrence of relapses [45]. Over 24 months, C-ANCA rose in 20 out of 58 patients. Nine patients were randomly assigned to receive a 9-month course of cyclophosphamide and a 3-month course of steroids at the time of the C-ANCA rise. Six of the 11 untreated patients relapsed within 3 months of the C-ANCA rise and three of the remaining five patients relapsed after 3 months during long-term follow-up. There were no early or late relapses in patients randomized for treatment. Furthermore, patients randomized for treatment based on an ANCA rise used less cyclophosphamide and steroids than the patients randomized for not being treated at the time of a rise.

In our recent study, we showed that measuring ANCA by ELISA is superior to measuring ANCA by IIF for the prediction of an ensuing relapse [32]. This implicates that treatment based on rises in ANCA as measured by ELISA could be more useful than treatment based on IIF titers. However, starting treatment with cyclophosphamide and steroids in patients with an ANCA rise exposes a number of patients to the unnecessary risk of drug-related morbidity since ANCA rises are not always followed by a relapse. Another important drawback of preventive treatment is that the time between an ANCA rise and a relapse is very variable. To address the question whether ANCA based treatment is beneficial, we recently started a large multi-center randomized study in which we evaluate whether treatment with a 9-month course of azathioprine and a 4.5-month course of steroids based on rises in ANCA levels as measured by ELISA is efficacious in preventing relapses in patients with Wegener's granulomatosis, and whether this prophylactic therapy outweighs the risk of unnecessary exposure to immunosuppressive drugs in some patients.

Prevention of relapses by anti-bacterial directed treatment

Several anecdotal reports have noted beneficial results on sulphamethoxazole-trimethoprim (co-trimoxazole) in the treatment of refractionary Wegener's granulo-

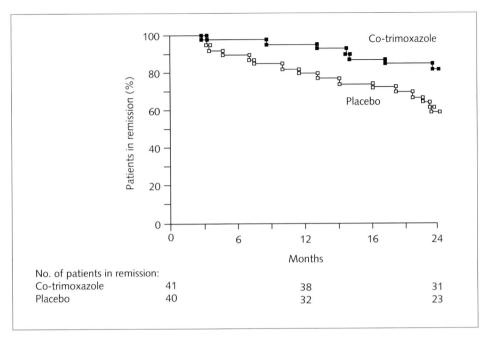

Figure 5
Disease free interval (vertical axis) counted from the start of the study medication in patients with Wegener's granulomatosis treated with co-trimoxazole (■, n = 41) or placebo (□, n = 40) during 24 months. The difference in disease free interval of patients allocated to co-tri-moxazole as compared to placebo is statistically significant by log rank test at 24 months (relative risk 0.40, 95 percent confidence interval, 0.17 to 0.98), but not at 36 months (relative risk 0.55, 95 percent confidence interval, 0.27 to 1.14) and 48 months (relative risk 0.63, 95 percent confidence interval, 0.32 to 1.24). The numbers above the horizontal axis indicate the number of patients disease free at risk at 12, 24, 36, and 48 months in the group allocated to co-trimoxazole (upper number) and placebo (lower number). Reprinted from [30] with permission of the publisher.

matosis, or limited Wegener's granulomatosis localized to the respiratory tract [58–61]. In a controlled prospective study, we demonstrated that prolonged prophylactic treatment with co-trimoxazole (800 mg sulphamethoxazole/160 mg trimethoprim) twice daily for 24 months leads to a reduced incidence of relapses as compared to placebo treatment in patients with Wegener's granulomatosis in whom remission is induced with cyclophosphamide and steroids (Fig. 5) [30]. Based on an intention to treat analysis, 82% of the patients remained relapse free with co-trimoxazole as compared to 60% with placebo. Adjusted for the only other factor found to be predictive of relapse, a positive ANCA titer at the start of the study, the relative risk for a relapse was 0.32 with co-trimoxazole treatment (95% confidence interval, 0.13–0.79). Furthermore, chronic co-trimoxazole treatment resulted in a significant reduction in the number of respiratory and non-respiratory infections. Finally, co-trimoxazole provides prophylaxis against infections with *Pneumocystis carinii*, which has been reported to be one of the most frequent and serious opportunistic infections during immunosuppressive therapy for Wegener's granulomatosis [62].

How co-trimoxazole exerts its beneficial effect on Wegener's granulomatosis is presently unclear. It is tempting to postulate that co-trimoxazole reduces the frequency of relapses by eliminating or suppressing the presence of *S. aureus* in the upper airways. Another possibility is that co-trimoxazole exerts anti-inflammatory effects and that the beneficial effects of this drug are not disease specific [63]. To further study this issue, a randomized controlled study has recently started in which intermittent use of mupirocine nasal ointment, which is an effective eradicator of nasal *S. aureus* carriage, is evaluated as maintenance therapy in Wegener's granulomatosis (MUPIBAC) [11].

A drawback of co-trimoxazole treatment is that about 20% of patients cannot tolerate this therapy due to adverse effects [30]. The adverse effects of co-trimoxazole treatment, however, are generally mild and fully reversible, and occur within the first few months after treatment has been started. Severe adverse effects have, however, been described [64]. Additionally, a substantial proportion of patients will not develop relapses of the disease, not even after prolonged follow-up. Overall, co-trimoxazole treatment reduces the absolute risk for a relapse during a 2-year follow-up period by 22%. This means that five patients (95% confidence interval, 3–31) have to be treated with co-trimoxazole for 24 months to prevent one relapse [65]. Thus, many patients will be unnecessarily exposed to long-term co-trimoxazole treatment. Furthermore, it is at present not known whether co-trimoxazole is also effective if used for longer periods than 24 months. Further studies are needed to address the issue of which patients are the best candidates for co-trimoxazole maintenance treatment.

Conclusion

Relapses occur in more than 50% of patients with ANCA associated vasculitis during follow-up. Within the spectrum of these vasculitides, relapses seem to occur more frequently in patients with Wegener's granulomatosis than in other forms of vasculitis. Nasal carriage of *S. aureus* is an important risk factor for relapses in Wegener's granulomatosis. Prolonged prophylactic treatment with co-trimoxazole results in a reduced incidence of relapses in these patients. The second risk factor for a relapse that has been identified is ANCA. Persistence of ANCA or the reappearance of ANCA are important risk factors for the development of a relapse. In addition, rising ANCA levels are associated with recurrence of the disease in many cases.

Theoretically, quantification of ANCA can be used as a therapeutic guideline in antibody directed treatment of patients with ANCA associated vasculitis. ANCA levels may either be used to institute "pre-emptive" therapy, or to adopt an approach in which reductions of immunosuppressive treatment are postponed in those patients who remain ANCA positive. At present, too few studies have been performed to draw any conclusion about whether one of these approaches should be used. Therefore, it is advised to use serial measurement of ANCA levels as an adjunctive to closely monitor patients for signs of disease relapse.

References

1   Fauci AS, Haynes B, Katz P (1978) The spectrum of vasculitis: clinical, pathologic, immunologic and therapeutic considerations. *Ann Intern Med* 89: 660–676

2   Fauci AS, Haynes BF, Katz P, Wolff SM (1983) Wegener's granulomatosis: prospective clinical and therapeutic experience with 85 patients for 21 years. *Ann Intern Med* 98: 76–85

3   Andrassy K, Erb A, Koderisch J, Waldherr R, Ritz E (1991) Wegener's granulomatosis with renal involvement: patient survival and correlations between initial renal function, renal histology, therapy and renal outcome. *Clin Nephrol* 35: 139–147

4   Hoffman GS, Kerr GS, Leavitt RY, Hallahan CW, Lebovics RS, Travis WD, Rottem M, Fauci AS (1992) Wegener Granulomatosis: An Analysis of 158 patients. *Ann Int Med* 116: 488–498

5   Gaskin G, Pusey CD (1992) Systemic vasculitis. In: JS Cameon, AM Davison, J Grünfeld, DNS Kerr, E Rits (eds): *Oxford textbook of clinical nephrology*. Oxford University Press, Oxford, 612–636

6   Balow JE, Fauci AS (1993) Vasculitic diseases of the kidney, polyarteritis, Wegener's granulomatosis, necrotizing and crescentic glomerulonephritis, and other disorders. In: RW Schrier, CW Gottschalk (eds): *Diseases of the kidney*. 5th Edition. Little, Brown and Company, Boston, 2095–2117

7   Stillwell TJ, Benson RC Jr, DeRemee RA, McDonald TJ, Weiland LH (1988) Cyclophosphamide-induced bladder toxicity in Wegener's granulomatosis. *Arthritis Rheum* 31: 465–470

8   Radis CD, Kahl LE, Baker GL, Wasko MC, Cash JM, Gallatin A, Stolzer BL, Agarwal AK, Medsger TA Jr, Kwoh CK (1995) Effects of cyclophosphamide on the development of malignancy and on long-term survival of patients with rheumatoid arthritis. A 20-year followup study. *Arthritis Rheum* 38: 1120–1127

9   Bouroncle BA, Smith EJ, Cuppage FE (1967) Treatment of Wegener's granulomatosis with Imuran. *Am J Med* 42: 314–318

10 Norton WL, Suki W, Strunk S (1968) Combined corticosteroid and azathioprine therapy in 2 patients with Wegener's granulomatosis. *Arch Intern Med* 121: 554–560

11 Jayne DR, Rasmussen N (1997) Treatment of antineutrophil cytoplasm autoantibody-

associated systemic vasculitis: initiatives of the European Community Systemic Vasculitis Clinical Trials Study Group. *Mayo Clin Proc* 72: 737–747

12   Jayne D (2000) Evidence-based treatment of systemic vasculitis. *Rheumatology* (Oxford) 39: 585–595

13   Jayne D Gaskin G (2000) Randomized trial of cyclophosphamide *versus* azathioprine during remission in ANCA associated systemic vasculitis (CYCAZAREM). *Clin Exp Immunol* 120 (Suppl 1): 53

14   de Groot K, Reinhold-Keller E, Tatsis E, Paulsen J, Heller M, Nolle B, Gross WL (1996) Therapy for the maintenance of remission in sixty-five patients with generalized Wegener's granulomatosis. Methotrexate *versus* trimethoprim/sulfamethoxazole. *Arthritis Rheum* 39: 2052–2061

15   Haubitz M, Koch KM, Brunkhorst R (1998) Cyclosporin for the prevention of disease reactivation in relapsing ANCA-associated vasculitis. *Nephrol Dial Transplant* 13: 2074–2076

16   Nowack R, Gobel U, Klooker P, Hergesell O, Andrassy K, van der Woude FJ (1999) Mycophenolate mofetil for maintenance therapy of Wegener's granulomatosis and microscopic polyangiitis: a pilot study in 11 patients with renal involvement. *J Am Soc Nephrol* 10: 1965–1971

17   Exley AR, Carruthers DM, Luqmani RA, Kitas GD, Gordon C, Janssen BA, Savage CO, Bacon PA (1997) Damage occurs early in systemic vasculitis and is an index of outcome. *Q J Med* 90: 391–399

18   Reinhold-Keller E, Kekow J, Schnabel A, Schmitt WH, Heller M, Beigel A, Duncker G, Gross WL (1994) Influence of disease manifestation and antineutrophil cytoplasmic antibody titer on the response to pulse cyclophosphamide therapy in patients with Wegener's granulomatosis. *Arthritis Rheum* 37: 919–924

19   Kallenberg CG, Cohen Tervaert JW, Stegeman CA (1990) Criteria for disease activity in Wegener's granulomatosis: a requirement for longitudinal clinical studies. *APMIS Suppl* 19: 37–39

20   Luqmani RA, Bacon PA, Moots RJ, Janssen BA, Pall A, Emery P, Savage C, Adu D (1994) Birmingham Vasculitis Activity Score (BVAS) in systemic necrotizing vasculitis. *Q J Med* 87: 671–678

21   Whiting-O'Keefe QE, Stone JH, Hellmann DB (1999) Validity of a vasculitis activity index for systemic necrotizing vasculitis. *Arthritis Rheum* 42: 2365–2371

22   Gordon M, Luqmani RA, Adu D, Greaves I, Richards N, Michael J, Emery P, Howie AJ, Bacon PA (1993) Relapses in patients with a systemic vasculitis. *Q J Med* 86: 779–789

23   Davenport A, Lock RJ, Wallington T (1995) Clinical significance of the serial measurement of autoantibodies to neutrophil cytoplasm using a standard indirect immunofluorescence test. *Am J Nephrol* 15: 201–207

24   Guillevin L, Cohen P, Gayraud M, Lhote F, Jarrousse B, Casassus P (1999) Churg-Strauss syndrome. Clinical study and long-term follow-up of 96 patients. *Medicine* (Baltimore) 78: 26–37

25   Kyndt X, Reumaux D, Bridoux F, Tribout B, Bataille P, Hachulla E, Hatron PY,

Duthilleul P, Vanhille P (1999) Serial measurements of antineutrophil cytoplasmic autoantibodies in patients with systemic vasculitis. *Am J Med* 106: 527–533

26   Reinhold-Keller E, Beuge N, Latza U, de Groot K, Rudert H, Nolle B, Heller M, Gross WL (2000) An interdisciplinary approach to the care of patients with Wegener's granulomatosis: long-term outcome in 155 patients. *Arthritis Rheum* 43: 1021–1032

27   Cohen Tervaert JW, van der Woude FJ, Fauci AS, Ambrus JL, Velosa J, Keane WF, Meijer S, van der Giessen M, The TH, van der Hem GK et al (1989) Association Between Active Wegener's Granulomatosis and Anticytoplasmic Antibodies. *Arch Intern Med* 149: 2461–2465

28   Stegeman CA, Cohen Tervaert JW, Sluiter WJ, Manson WL, de Jong PE, Kallenberg CG (1994) Association of chronic nasal carriage of Staphylococcus aureus and higher relapse rates in Wegener granulomatosis. *Ann Intern Med* 120: 12–17

29   Nachman PH, Hogan SL, Jennette JC, Falk RJ (1996) Treatment response and relapse in antineutrophil cytoplasmic autoantibody-associated microscopic polyangiitis and glomerulonephritis. *J Am Soc Nephrol* 7:33–9

30   Stegeman CA, Cohen Tervaert JW, de Jong PE, CG Kallenberg (1996) Trimethoprim-sulfamethoxazole (co-trimoxazole) for the prevention of relapses of Wegener's Granulomatosis. *N Engl J Med* 335: 16–20

31   Westman KW, Bygren PG, Olsson H, Ranstam J, Wieslander J (1998) Relapse rate, renal survival, and cancer morbidity in patients with Wegener's granulomatosis or microscopic polyangiitis with renal involvement. *J Am Soc Nephrol* 9: 842–852

32   Boomsma MM, Stegeman CA, Leij van der MJ, Oost W, Hermans J, Kallenberg CGM, Limburg PC, Cohen Tervaert JW (2000) Prediction of relapses in Wegener's granulomatosis by measurement of Anti Neutrophil Cytoplasmic Antibody levels; a prospective study. *Arthritis Rheum* 43: 2025–2033

33   Kerr GS, Fleisher TA, Hallahan CW, Leavitt RY, Fauci AS, Hoffman GS (1993) Limited prognostic value of changes in antineutrophil cytoplasmic antibody titer in patients with Wegener's granulomatosis. *Arthritis Rheum* 36: 365–371

34   De'Oliviera J, Gaskin G, Dash A, Rees AJ, Pusey CD (1995) Relationship between disease activity and anti-neutrophil cytoplasmic antibody concentration in long-term management of systemic vasculitis. *Am J Kidney Dis* 25: 380–389

35   Geffriaud-Ricouard C, Noel LH, Chauveau D, Houhou S, Grunfeld JP, Lesavre P (1993) Clinical spectrum associated with ANCA of defined antigen specificities in 98 selected patients. *Clin Nephrol* 39: 125–136

36   Franssen C, Gans R, Kallenberg C, Hageluken C, Hoorntje S (1998) Disease spectrum of patients with antineutrophil cytoplasmic autoantibodies of defined specificity: distinct differences between patients with anti-proteinase 3 and anti-myeloperoxidase autoantibodies. *J Intern Med* 244: 209–216

37   Davies DJ, Moran JE, Niall JF, Ryan GB (1982) Segmental necrotising glomerulonephritis with antineutrophil antibody: possible arbovirus aetiology? *Br Med J (Clin Res Ed)* 285: 606

38   van der Woude FJ, Rasmussen N, Lobatto S, Wiik A, Permin H, van Es LA, van der

Giessen M, van der Hem GK, The TH (1985) Autoantibodies against neutrophils and monocytes: tool for diagnosis and marker of disease activity in Wegener's granulomatosis. *Lancet* 1: 425–429

39   Falk RJ, Jennette JC (1988) Anti-neutrophil cytoplasmic autoantibodies with specificity for myeloperoxidase in patients with systemic vasculitis and idiopathic necrotizing and crescentic glomerulonephritis. *N Engl J Med* 318: 1651–1657

40   Cohen Tervaert JW, Goldschmeding R, Elema JD, Limburg PC, van der Giessen M, Huitema MG, Koolen MI, Hene RJ, The TH, van der Hem GK, et al (1990) Association of autoantibodies to myeloperoxidase with different forms of vasculitis. *Arthritis Rheum* 33: 1264–1272

41   Franssen CF, Stegeman CA, Kallenberg CG, Gans RO, De Jong PE, Hoorntje SJ, Tervaert JW (2000) Antiproteinase 3- and antimyeloperoxidase-associated vasculitis. *Kidney Int* 57: 2195–2206

42   Jayne DR, Gaskin G, Pusey CD, Lockwood CM (1995) ANCA and predicting relapse in systemic vasculitis. *Q J Med* 88: 127–133

43   Franssen CF, Stegeman CA, Oost-Kort WW, Kallenberg CG, Limburg PC, Tiebosch A, De Jong PE, Cohen Tervaert JW (1998) Determinants of renal outcome in anti-myeloperoxidase-associated necrotizing crescentic glomerulonephritis. *J Am Soc Nephrol* 9: 1915–1923

44   Egner W, Chapel HM (1990) Titration of antibodies against neutrophil cytoplasmic antigens is useful in monitoring disease activity in systemic vasculitides. *Clin Exp Immunol* 82: 244–249

45   Cohen Tervaert JW, Huitema MG, Hené RJ, Sluiter WJ, The TH, van der Hem GK, Kallenberg CG (1990) Prevention of relapses in Wegener's Granulomatosis by treatment based on antineutrophil cytoplasmic antibody titre. *Lancet* 336: 706–711

46   Chan TM, Frampton G, Jayne DR, Perry GJ, Lockwood CM, Cameron JS (1993) Clinical significance of anti-endothelial cell antibodies in systemic vasculitis: a longitudinal study comparing anti-endothelial cell antibodies and anti-neutrophil cytoplasm antibodies. *Am J Kidney Dis* 22: 387–392

47   Hagen EC, Andrassy K, Chernok E, Daha MR, Gaskin G, Gross W, Lesavre P, Ludemann J, Pusey CD, Rasmussen N et al (1993) The value of indirect immunofluorescence and solid phase techniques for ANCA detection. A report on the first phase of an international cooperative study on the standardization of ANCA assays. EEC/BCR Group for ANCA Assay Standardization. *J Immunol Methods* 159: 1–16

48   Mulder AH, Stegeman CA, Kallenberg CG (1995) Activation of granulocytes by anti-neutrophil cytoplasmic antibodies (ANCA) in Wegener's granulomatosis: a predominant role for the IgG3 subclass of ANCA. *Clin Exp Immunol* 101: 227–232

49   Cohen Tervaert JW, Mulder AHL, Kallenberg CGM, Stegeman CA (1994) Measurement of IgG3 of anti-proteinase 3 antibodies to neutrophil cytoplasm is useful in monitoring disease activity in Wegener's granulomatosis. *J Am Soc Nephrol* 5: 828

50   van de Wiel BA, Dolman KM, van der Meer-Gerritsen CH, Hack CE, von dem Borne

AE, Goldschmeding R (1992) Interference of Wegener's granulomatosis autoantibodies with neutrophil Proteinase 3 activity. *Clin Exp Immunol* 90: 409–414

51 Dolman KM, Stegeman CA, van de Wiel BA, Hack CE, von dem Borne AE, Kallenberg CG, Goldschmeding R (1993) Relevance of classic anti-neutrophil cytoplasmic autoantibody (C-ANCA)-mediated inhibition of proteinase 3-alpha 1-antitrypsin complexation to disease activity in Wegener's granulomatosis. *Clin Exp Immunol* 93: 405–410

52 Daouk GH, Palsson R, Arnaout MA (1995) Inhibition of proteinase 3 by ANCA and its correlation with disease activity in Wegener's granulomatosis. *Kidney Int* 47: 1528–1536

53 Pinching AJ, Rees AJ, Pussell BA, Lockwood CM, Mitchison RS, Peters DK (1980) Relapses in Wegener's granulomatosis: the role of infection. *Br Med J* 281: 836–838

54 Ronco P, Verroust P, Mignon F, Kourilsky O, Vanhille P, Meyrier A, Mery JP, Morel-Maroger L (1983) Immunopathological studies of polyarteritis nodosa and Wegener's granulomatosis: a report of 43 patients with 51 renal biopsies. *Q J Med* 52: 212–223

55 Gadola S, Sahly H, Reinhold-Keller E, Hellmich B, Paulsen J, Gross WL (1998) Nasal carriage of staphylococcus aureus and association with disease activity in Wegener's granulomatosis [Abstract] *Clin Exp Immunol* 112 (Suppl 1): 23

56 Hogan SL, Nachman PH, Jennette JC, Falk RJ (1998) Predictors of relapse in ANCA small vessel vasculitis [Abstract] *Clin Exp Immunol* 112 (Suppl 1): 23

57 Dijstelbloem HM, Scheepers RH, Oost WW, Stegeman CA, van der Pol WL, Sluiter WJ, Kallenberg CG, van de Winkel JG, Tervaert JW (1999) Fcgamma receptor polymorphisms in Wegener's granulomatosis: risk factors for disease relapse. *Arthritis Rheum* 42: 1823–1827

58 DeRemee RA, McDonald TJ, Weiland LH (1985) Wegener's granulomatosis: observations on treatment with antimicrobial agents. *Mayo Clin Proc* 60: 27–32

59 DeRemee RA (1988) The treatment of Wegener's granulomatosis with trimethoprim / sulfamethoxazole: illusion or vision? *Arthritis Rheum* 31: 1068–1074

60 Israel HL (1988) Sulfamethoxazole-trimethoprim therapy for Wegener's granulomatosis. *Arch Intern Med* 148: 2293–2295

61 Valeriano-Marcet J, Spiera H (1991) Treatment of Wegener's granulomatosis with sulfamethoxazole-trimethoprim. *Arch Intern Med* 151: 1649–1652

62 Ognibene FP, Shelhamer JH, Hoffman GS, Kerr GS, Reda D, Fauci AS, Leavitt RY (1995) Pneumocystis carinii pneumonia: a major complication of immunosuppressive therapy in patients with Wegener's granulomatosis. *Am J Respir Crit Care Med* 151: 795–799

63 Roberts DE, Curd JG (1990) Sulfonamides as antiinflammatory agents in the treatment of Wegener's granulomatosis. *Arthritis Rheum* 33: 1590–1593

64 Rubin RH, Swartz MN (1980) Trimethoprim-sulfamethoxazole. *N Engl J Med* 303: 426–432

65 Stegeman CA, Cohen Tervaert JW, Kallenberg CG (1997) Co-trimoxazole and Wegener's granulomatosis: more than a coincidence? *Nephrol Dial Transplant* 12: 652–655

Index

The PIR-Series
Progress in Inflammation Research

Homepage: http://www.birkhauser.ch

Up-to-date information on the latest developments in the pathology, mechanisms and therapy of inflammatory disease are provided in this monograph series. Areas covered include vascular responses, skin inflammation, pain, neuroinflammation, arthritis cartilage and bone, airways inflammation and asthma, allergy, cytokines and inflammatory mediators, cell signalling, and recent advances in drug therapy. Each volume is edited by acknowledged experts providing succinct overviews on specific topics intended to inform and explain. The series is of interest to academic and industrial biomedical researchers, drug development personnel and rheumatologists, allergists, pathologists, dermatologists and other clinicians requiring regular scientific updates.

Available volumes:
T Cells in Arthritis, P. Miossec, W. van den Berg, G. Firestein (Editors), 1998
Chemokines and Skin, E. Kownatzki, J. Norgauer (Editors), 1998
Medicinal Fatty Acids, J. Kremer (Editor), 1998
Inducible Enzymes in the Inflammatory Response, D.A. Willoughby, A. Tomlinson (Editors), 1999
Cytokines in Severe Sepsis and Septic Shock, H. Redl, G. Schlag (Editors), 1999
Fatty Acids and Inflammatory Skin Diseases, J.-M. Schröder (Editor), 1999
Immunomodulatory Agents from Plants, H. Wagner (Editor), 1999
Cytokines and Pain, L. Watkins, S. Maier (Editors), 1999
In Vivo *Models of Inflammation*, D. Morgan, L. Marshall (Editors), 1999
Pain and Neurogenic Inflammation, S.D. Brain, P. Moore (Editors), 1999
Anti-Inflammatory Drugs in Asthma, A.P. Sampson, M.K. Church (Editors), 1999
Novel Inhibitors of Leukotrienes, G. Folco, B. Samuelsson, R.C. Murphy (Editors), 1999
Vascular Adhesion Molecules and Inflammation, J.D. Pearson (Editor), 1999
Metalloproteinases as Targets for Anti-Inflammatory Drugs, K.M.K. Bottomley, D. Bradshaw, J.S. Nixon (Editors), 1999
Free Radicals and Inflammation, P.G. Winyard, D.R. Blake, C.H. Evans (Editors), 1999
Gene Therapy in Inflammatory Diseases, C.H. Evans, P. Robbins (Editors), 2000
New Cytokines as Potential Drugs, S. K. Narula, R. Coffmann (Editors), 2000
High Throughput Screening for Novel Anti-inflammatories, M. Kahn (Editor), 2000
Immunology and Drug Therapy of Atopic Skin Diseases, C.A.F. Bruijnzeel-Komen, E.F. Knol (Editors), 2000
Novel Cytokine Inhibitors, G.A. Higgs, B. Henderson (Editors), 2000
Inflammatory Processes. Molecular Mechanisms and Therapeutic Opportunities, L.G. Letts, D.W. Morgan (Editors), 2000

Cellular Mechanisms in Airways Inflammation, C. Page, K. Banner, D. Spina (Editors), 2000
Inflammatory and Infectious Basis of Atherosclerosis, J.L. Mehta (Editor), 2001
Muscarinic Receptors in Airways Diseases, J. Zaagsma, H. Meurs, A.F. Roffel (Editors), 2001
TGF-β and Related Cytokines in Inflammation, S.N. Breit, S. Wahl (Editors), 2001
Nitric Oxide and Inflammation, D. Salvemini, T.R. Billiar, Y. Vodovotz (Editors), 2001
Neuroinflammatory Mechanisms in Alzheimer's Disease. Basic and Clinical Research, J. Rogers (Editor), 2001